"*Previvors* will truly be an asset to women and their families who face difficult decisions surrounding breast and ovarian cancer risk. Dina Roth Port does an excellent job communicating the issues and alternatives of this very emotional subject in a factual, well-referenced way. What an impressive book!"

—Leslie G. Ford, M.D., Associate Director for Clinical Research, Division of Cancer Prevention, National Cancer Institute, NIH

"*Previvors* is a perfect companion for anyone who faces being at high risk for cancer. Since the moment FORCE first coined the term 'previvor,' awareness has been growing. This book takes previvor awareness and education to the next level."

—Sue Friedman, Founder and Executive Director, FORCE

"The women featured in *Previvors* are heroes for sharing their stories, and the book will no doubt save many lives. Dina Roth Port has delivered a brilliant resource that will guide women through the genetic revolution with knowledge, and perhaps even more important, hope."

—Geralyn Lucas, author of *Why I Wore Lipstick to My Mastectomy*

"*Previvors* is thoughtful and insightful, and an essential guide for countless women who need to learn about their risk for breast cancer and what they can do about it. The five women's stories paint a vivid picture of what it's like to be a previvor, while the book is also packed with sound research and advice. I finally have a book I can recommend to my patients who have breast cancer in their families."

—Christy Russell, M.D., national board member of the American Cancer Society, Codirector, University of Southern California/Norris Lee Breast Center

"*Previvors* is truly a gift to all women who are at high risk for breast and ovarian cancer. Presented in an easy-to-digest fashion and sprinkled with the inspiring stories of those who have already endured the journey, this book is a long-awaited essential tool."

—Lindsay Avner, Founder and Executive Director, Bright Pink

"Dina Roth Port's *Previvors* is a superb practical guide for navigating the uncharted waters of the breast cancer gene. Brava to Dina for supplying much-needed information in this engaging book."

—Jessica Queller, author of *Pretty Is What Changes*

"For women with a high risk of breast cancer, navigating the myriad decisions to be made about genetic testing, cancer screening, and risk-reducing surgeries can be overwhelming. *Previvors* provides valuable, unbiased information. . . . It is a must-read for women at risk, their relatives and friends!"

—Angela Trepanier, past President, National Society of Genetic Counselors

"When I was considering my preventive mastectomy, I searched for information to help me through the confusing, emotional process of weighing my options and figuring out how to protect myself. *Previvors* is the book I wished I had then. I urge women who are facing their cancer risk to pick up a copy of this informative guide."

—René Syler, TV personality and author of *Good-Enough Mother*

"Complete with a tremendous wealth of information and very relatable true stories, this is a book every previvor should read!"

—Rebecca Sutphen, M.D., former Director of Clinical Genetics, Moffitt Cancer Center

"Dina Roth Port has created an invaluable resource for women with a family history of cancer. This guide provides a clear explanation of the genetic evaluation and testing process, as well as management options for women with a high risk for breast cancer. I highly recommend the book for my patients seeking reliable information on this topic."

—Therese Bevers, M.D., Medical Director, Cancer Prevention Center
at M. D. Anderson Cancer Center

"*Previvors* is a desperately needed resource for women who are trying to make decisions about their high-risk status. The book spells out the various imaging tests that are available, along with their benefits and weaknesses, and it will help many women sort through such options."

—Kathryn Evers, M.D., Director of Breast Imaging, Fox Chase Cancer Center

"*Previvors* is an enjoyable and educational read that puts readers in touch with the emotional and physical side of having a high risk for someday developing breast cancer."

—Lillie D. Shockney, R.N., B.S., MAS, Johns Hopkins Avon Foundation Breast Center

previvors

Dina Roth Port

Includes the stories of
Suzanne Citere, Rori Clark,
Lisa Marton, Amy Rosenthal,
and Mayde Wiener

previvors

FACING THE BREAST CANCER GENE
AND MAKING LIFE-CHANGING DECISIONS

AVERY

a member of Penguin Group (USA) Inc.

New York

Published by the Penguin Group

Penguin Group (USA) Inc., 375 Hudson Street, New York, New York 10014, USA · Penguin Group (Canada), 90 Eglinton Avenue East, Suite 700, Toronto, Ontario M4P 2Y3, Canada (a division of Pearson Penguin Canada Inc.) · Penguin Books Ltd, 80 Strand, London WC2R 0RL, England · Penguin Ireland, 25 St Stephen's Green, Dublin 2, Ireland (a division of Penguin Books Ltd) · Penguin Group (Australia), 250 Camberwell Road, Camberwell, Victoria 3124, Australia (a division of Pearson Australia Group Pty Ltd) · Penguin Books India Pvt Ltd, 11 Community Centre, Panchsheel Park, New Delhi-110 017, India · Penguin Group (NZ), 67 Apollo Drive, Rosedale, North Shore 0632, New Zealand (a division of Pearson New Zealand Ltd) · Penguin Books (South Africa) (Pty) Ltd, 24 Sturdee Avenue, Rosebank, Johannesburg 2196, South Africa

Penguin Books Ltd, Registered Offices: 80 Strand, London WC2R 0RL, England

Most Avery books are available at special quantity discounts for bulk purchase for sales promotions, premiums, fund-raising, and educational needs. Special books or book excerpts also can be created to fit specific needs. For details, write Penguin Group (USA) Inc. Special Markets, 375 Hudson Street, New York, NY 10014.

Library of Congress Cataloging-in-Publication Data

Port, Dina Roth.
Previvors: facing the breast cancer gene and making life-changing decisions / Dina Roth Port.
p.   cm.
"Includes the stories of Suzanne Citere, Rori Clark, Lisa Marton, Amy Rosenthal, and Mayde Wiener."
ISBN 978-1-58333-405-8
1. Breast—Cancer—Genetic aspects.   2. Breast—Cancer—Risk factors.
3. Breast—Cancer—Prevention.   4. Mastectomy.   I. Title.
RC280.B8P66 2010.   2010023026
616.99'499—dc22

Printed in the United States of America
1 3 5 7 9 10 8 6 4 2

BOOK DESIGN BY NICOLE LAROCHE

Neither the publisher nor the author is engaged in rendering professional advice or services to the individual reader. The ideas, procedures, and suggestions contained in this book are not intended as a substitute for consulting with your physician. All matters regarding your health require medical supervision. Neither the author nor the publisher shall be liable or responsible for any loss or damage allegedly arising from any information or suggestion in this book.

This publication is designed to provide accurate and authoritative information in regard to the subject matter covered. It is sold with the understanding that the publisher is not engaged in rendering legal, accounting, or other professional services. If you require legal advice or other expert assistance, you should seek the services of a competent professional.

Some names and identifying characteristics have been changed to protect the privacy of the individuals involved.

While the author has made every effort to provide accurate telephone numbers and Internet addresses at the time of publication, neither the publisher nor the author assumes any responsibility for errors, or for changes that occur after publication. Further, the publisher does not have any control over and does not assume any responsibility for author or third-party websites or their content.

To those we have lost to cancer.

To those we have watched suffer.

And to those we hope never will.

contents

foreword

During the past two decades, the pace of genetic discovery and medical progress in cancer genetics has been rapid. For many of us who were working in this field in the early 1990s, it has been startling to participate in and witness the expansion of knowledge applied to families affected by the more than fifty inherited genetic syndromes that increase risk for cancers of the breast, ovary, colon, prostate, and other organs. These scientific and medical advances have been accompanied by an equally rapid set of social and ethical accommodations. A young woman reading *Previvors* today would be surprised to learn that this account of the sagas of Lisa, Mayde, Amy, Rori, and Suzanne would have been called scientifically fictitious, as well as socially stigmatizing, less than two decades ago.

As great as the scientific challenges, a significant obstacle to raising awareness and empowering women at risk for breast cancer was the perceived threat of social stigma. Before the passage of the Genetic Information Nondiscrimination Act in 2008, a powerful and inspiring story like the one in *Previvors* would have been more difficult to document. Such a moving narrative about women at hereditary risk for breast cancer, speaking openly and referring to their personal histories, would have been viewed by some as a potential risk. While the threat of genetic discrimination by health insurers or employers is now effectively removed, the perception of stigma remains in some communities. When my team discovered the most common BRCA2 mutation in 1996, and linked it to people of Ashkenazi Jewish ancestry, many were concerned about "group stigmatization" of those members of geographical and ethnic cohorts at higher risk for hereditary diseases. It has taken us the better part of a decade to refocus these groups to recognize the extraordinary opportunities afforded by these discoveries as a means for more effective cancer prevention and early detection.

The fundamental scientific and medical challenge during this period stemmed from the question "What is the point of genetic testing if nothing can be done about it?" At the time, Dr. Francis Collins, then head of the U.S. Human Genome Project, and now head of the National Institutes of Health, cited this aphorism: "It is but sorrow to be wise when wisdom profits not." This statement from Sophocles was seen by some as encouraging women to think twice about a genetic test with no proven means for prevention or early detection. Contained in the pages of *Previvors* is a concise distillation of the range of options for medical and surgical screening and prevention that are now available to women who are at greatest risk for breast cancer. Risk-reducing surgery of the ovaries, for example, was shown by our group, and confirmed by others, to decrease the burden of both breast and ovarian cancer in families with BRCA mutations. In other cases, a universal consensus of experts has not emerged as far as the preferred option. One such example is the effectiveness of surveillance using magnetic resonance imaging (MRI) of the breast, compared with preventative bilateral mastectomy. To guide this choice, individual decisions need to be made. In a clear style that is cast in human terms that are also scientifically accurate, Dina Roth Port has provided families with an extraordinary resource. She has created an annotated and informed map of the many paths available after cancer genetic testing.

Previvors is thus an invaluable resource for women and families at the vanguard of the "genetic revolution" in cancer medicine. It also offers inspiration for the scientists and humanists who seek to responsibly translate these scientific discoveries into improved health care for all.

KENNETH OFFIT, M.D., MPH

Chief, Clinical Genetics Service; Vice Chairman, Academic Affairs,

Department of Medicine; and Vice Chairman, Program in Cancer Prevention

and Population Research, Memorial Sloan-Kettering Cancer Center

Member, Cancer Biology and Genetics Program (joint), Sloan-Kettering Institute

Professor of Medicine and Public Health, Weill Cornell Medical College of Cornell University

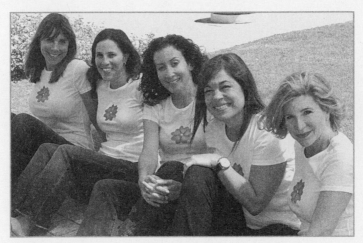

Rori, Amy, Lisa, Suzanne, and Mayde

(From left to right)

previvors

previvors

Lisa never considered herself a prude, but she wasn't the type to go into a public restroom, take off her bra, and expose her breasts to a stranger. But that's just what this young mom did in a Dunkin' Donuts bathroom one Sunday afternoon. As her friend Mayde encouraged her, Lisa let a woman named Suzanne stare at her naked chest for several minutes. And while this was happening, two other women named Rori and Amy sat at a table and watched Lisa's preschooler nibble on chocolate-glazed Munchkins.

To an outsider, such an encounter might seem a bit depraved. In fact, it was anything but. Lisa was only doing what Amy and Mayde had done for her in a stir-fry restaurant a few months earlier—a "show-and-tell" of what reconstructed breasts look like after a mastectomy. It's an initiation of sorts: Someone who has had a mastectomy will go into a bathroom—in a person's home, Starbucks, McDonald's, you name it—and give a sneak preview to a woman who is considering one. Touching is often encouraged. Many breast cancer survivors perform these "show-and-tells," but Lisa, Mayde, Amy, and Rori were different. None of them had ever had cancer, but all had undergone mastectomies to prevent the disease they felt they were destined to get. Suzanne's same surgery was scheduled for two months later.

These women are previvors: people who have not had cancer but possess a predisposition to develop it. For some men and women, it means having a family history of breast cancer or other risk factors. For others, it also means testing positive for one of the breast cancer gene mutations. While many options exist for the vast number of breast cancer previvors alive today—from surveillance to prophylactic mastectomies—these five women ultimately chose the same path. It was the bond that initiated a special, unique friendship.

That spring day amid the French crullers and jelly donuts, these women from South Florida gathered for the first time. Mayde had met Suzanne when her daughter started tap lessons at Suzanne's dance studio. After learning that Suzanne's mother had died young from breast cancer, Mayde encouraged her to tackle her risk head-on and provided her with information on how to do so. Months later, when Suzanne started considering the prophylactic surgery, Mayde invited her to the impromptu get-together at Dunkin' Donuts to meet Lisa, Rori, and Amy, women she had met through FORCE (Facing Our Risk of Cancer Empowered), a nonprofit organization for women at risk for breast and ovarian cancer. They had all helped each other while weighing their options. Now it was their turn to help Suzanne.

For hours they talked about everything from what size cup they chose and why they kept their nipples to how their husbands reacted to their new breasts. They told stories about their mothers—all had battled cancer; a few of them lost the war. The energy between the five women was palpable. They felt deeply connected to one another, as though they had known each other forever.

It was an unlikely group of friends. At a glance, they are very different:

With short blond hair and funky glasses, Mayde looks like a quirky sophisticate who knows what she's talking about. And she does. She's smart as a whip and so knowledgeable about breast cancer you'd think she was an expert in the field. She does extensive research about everything in her life—from which schools her children attend to what kind of cell phone to buy—so that she can make the best possible decisions. Growing up, Mayde was "that" kid in high school—even though she was one of the youngest in her class, she was president of the honor society, salutatorian, and editor of her school newspaper. She also has an inborn need to help others—she volunteered at local hospitals as a teenager, and she eventually went to medical school and started her own podiatry practice. Now she's a stay-at-home mom who has made it her mission to guide other women who are first dealing with their risk for breast cancer. If it weren't for Mayde, the five women in this book never would have found each other.

Amy's the youngest and, checking in at just under five feet tall, she looks more youthful than her years. Her personality matches her appearance—she's bubbly, has a killer sense of humor, and is so outgoing she'll talk to anyone, anywhere. But she wouldn't admit to that—Amy appears unaware of her strengths and never boasts or brags. Trendy but reserved (she's the only one of the women who won't wear shirts that show off her new cleavage), she's a dedicated single mom who spends the little bit of "me time" she allows herself on the tennis courts. She's compassionate and easy to talk to, the kind of friend who will spend hours analyzing over and obsessing about anything. And Amy actually listens. If you tell her something that's bothering you, she'll call a few days later to follow up. However, when it comes to her own feelings—particularly about her family's history of breast cancer—she keeps them inside. She's quick to say, "I'm over it," though, in truth, she really isn't.

If you wanted to describe Suzanne in a few words, an "Italian girl from Brooklyn" would do the trick. With an athletic build and olive complexion, she's proud of her heritage and considers a slice from New York the only kind of pizza worth eating. Suzanne's the type of friend who'll tell it like it is. She's genuine, always speaks her mind, and doesn't take "no" for an answer. Her strength also comes from the fact that she grew up without a mother and had to fend for herself at a very young age. But along with her tough exterior, she wears her heart on her sleeve and will drop everything to help a loved one. She owns a dance studio for kids and spends half her day wiping noses, kissing foreheads, and nurturing little ballerinas before heading home to her own young daughter. Suzanne is also spontaneous and keeps a small suitcase packed in case she ever decides to take a last-minute trip. She has seen firsthand how fragile life can be and always tries to live with no regrets.

Rori is the "Little Miss Sunshine" of the group. She's someone you just can't help but love, with a smile that lights up the room and soft brown eyes that sparkle. On the one hand, she's a girly girl with a flair for fashion—she worked for a major designer for ten years and follows the latest trends. But also being completely laid-back, she's even more comfortable in stylish jeans and a T-shirt (paired with a great purse and sunglasses, of course). Rori is a hands-on type of person, especially when it comes to her kids, and she spends her days helping at their schools and then shuttling them to and from soccer, football, piano, and dance classes. Of all the women, Rori was the most attached to her breasts and had the hardest time making the decision to have the surgery. Also, though her family has seen its share of tragedy, she tries to block it all out. Instead, she remains a free spirit who believes in holistic living and finds inner peace by running, doing yoga, counting her blessings, and taking each day as it comes.

Lisa is a fireball, a true type-A go-getter. If you want a job done right, Lisa's the girl you can trust to come through for you. With long dark curls and a raspy voice, she has an infectious personality and is the type to walk into a party of strangers and know everyone by name when she leaves. People gravitate toward her because she has so much energy and is just fun to be around. Lisa is constantly on the go, BlackBerry in hand, making business deals one minute and play dates for her three kids the next. She's climbed her way to the top of almost every marketing company she's worked for and is always looking for her next project. She also loves exercising and finds her workouts to be the only time she "turns it all off." Lisa aims to find balance in her life and says that, especially after losing her mom, friends are an essential part of that equilibrium.

Despite their many differences, the five women were drawn together that day at Dunkin' Donuts, sharing a bond not even their husbands, children, or siblings could understand. They started meeting every few weeks for lunch, and in between would spend hours e-mailing, texting, and chatting on the phone. At first, they'd talk about their breasts, but then they'd move on to their kids, jobs, fashion—the typical topics any group of girlfriends might discuss.

The women felt so blessed to have each other, especially since women with an elevated risk for breast cancer have very few outlets besides FORCE and another national organization called Bright Pink. Sure, there are plenty of books for survivors of breast cancer, but almost none for women like them. They are part of a new generation of women who aim to beat cancer before it even strikes. That's why they decided that they needed to share their stories, not only with each other but also with the thousands, if not millions, of women who are in the same boat. It is our hope to provide these other pre-vivors with a comprehensive resource that will help guide them. In the end, many won't choose the same course of action these five women did, but they will all have to grapple with similar issues to figure out what's right for them. This is the book that Lisa, Mayde, Amy, Rori, and Suzanne wish had been available while they were making such agonizing decisions. It is the book they wish their mothers could have had.

living in fear

When Amy was a little girl, she used to think that someday she'd go to college, get married, and have kids. And then she'd get breast cancer. "I always figured breast cancer was just a way of life," she explains. "My Grandma Ada died from it right before I was born, and as I grew up I remember that my mother would be so nervous when she had her mammograms each year, acting as if cancer was inevitable. Then, when her results came back fine, I'd overhear her telling my father something like, 'Good news, I dodged the bullet again.' My mom was so convinced she'd get breast cancer that I assumed I'd just follow in her footsteps. As a child, I didn't quite know what that meant. But as I got older and learned what this illness could do to a person, it became terrifying."

Mayde also thought she'd get breast cancer someday. When she was seventeen, she watched her mom combat the disease, and later she started keeping a copy of her mother's pathology report tucked away in her underwear drawer. "I knew I was going to need it eventually," she says. "It was just a matter of time."

All diseases are scary, but for some reason breast cancer packs a particular punch. In fact, one survey showed that women fear this illness more than any other, even though cardiovascular disease claims more than ten times as many women's lives each year. Holly Priger-son, Ph.D., a psychiatry professor at Harvard Medical School and a psycho-oncologist at Dana-Farber Cancer Institute in Boston works with patients dealing with the psychological aspects of cancer. She says that fear of breast cancer is sometimes so powerful that people become paralyzed by it. "Whether from accounts in the media or first-hand experience, women often have a vivid image of breast cancer as a painful, debilitating, disfiguring disease that eventually attacks your vital organs and kills you," Dr. Prigerson says. "The truth is, breast cancer is usually *not* a death sentence. But it's still many women's worst nightmare."

That's especially the case for women who already know they have an elevated risk for getting the disease. They feel like they're looking into a crystal ball and seeing a horrifying future. Many have witnessed how breast cancer can destroy a person to the point that it deprives them of their dignity, their spirit, and eventually their life. The thought that that might also happen to them becomes unbearable.

how it begins

Suzanne remembers being two years old and waking up her mother, Nina, on Christmas morning to tell her that Santa Claus had left presents under the tree. That's the only memory she has of her mom. The following year, Nina found out she had terminal breast cancer. Two years later, on Suzanne's first day of kindergarten, she died. She was only forty-seven.

Fear of breast cancer doesn't just appear out of thin air. It stems from a source; there's a definitive point in time when it all begins. For some, that might be something as innocuous as reading a magazine story about a woman who battled the disease. For others, it's often watching a loved one actually suffer to the end with it.

After her mother's death, Suzanne's life changed drastically. "My dad worked seventy hours a week as a garment presser and would leave the house early in the morning and come home late at night," she says. "So my mom's sister, Aunt Lily, took care of me during the week and then I'd go home with my father on weekends.

"Growing up, I became extremely attached to my dad and was so afraid that he would also become sick and die. Often, in the middle of the night, I'd sneak into his room to check if he was still breathing. My dad rarely talked about my mom, but he never seemed to get over losing her. He became very withdrawn and, in a way, it was like I lost him, too. My sister and brother were ten and twenty years older than me, respectively, so they also weren't around for most of my child-hood. I was very lonely.

"If all of this had happened today, I probably would have gone to see a therapist," Suzanne continues. "But instead, my family and I relied on each other, our faith, and like most Italians, 'food therapy' to get through this difficult time. Every Sunday, Aunt Lily would start cook-ing the marinara sauce early in the morning while my grandmother would make pasta from scratch. Then in the afternoon my entire extended family would meet at Aunt Lily's and we'd feast on antipasti, pasta with meatballs and sausage, chicken or roast beef, and a salad. For dessert, we'd usually have my grandma's anisette-flavored cookies, plus other cakes and sweets. I really looked forward to those Sunday meals because everyone was so boisterous and animated, and we'd all just laugh and have fun together. But the rest of the week was sad for me because life at my aunt's house wasn't easy. My aunt and uncle took me in because they felt they had no choice, and they seemed resentful. They were nice to me, but I always felt like a burden.

"When I was a kid, people would often say, 'Oh, you poor thing. You lost your mother so young. That must have been so hard for you,'" adds Suzanne. "Truth be told, her death wasn't that difficult for me at the time. It's like telling someone who is blind from birth that they must miss not being able to see. I couldn't miss something I never really had. All I ever knew about my mom was from stories my dad's sister, Aunt Mary, and her husband, Uncle Sal, would tell me. When they'd see me getting worked up about something, they'd say, 'You're just like your mom.' Apparently she was a spitfire and an outspoken, liberated woman. She was a typical Italian mother—warm and loving, but strict. She was also the mom all the kids in the neighborhood wanted to have as their own, and the friend people always turned to for advice. Her death seemed to touch everyone in our community in Brooklyn. In fact, the line to get into her viewing at the funeral home stretched down the block, and afterward the service at the church was packed. But I never wanted to think about my mom too much— especially about how she died. I guess, like my dad, that was always my defense mechanism."

But as Suzanne grew older, her mother's history began to haunt her. "My mother got diagnosed with cancer at forty-five and I once read that I should start getting mammograms ten years before that," she says. "When I turned thirty-five, it was as if someone said to me, 'Okay, *now* you can start worrying.' Oddly enough, I never performed breast self-examinations because I was so petrified that I'd find something. Instead, I would have a mammogram every January and then bury my head in the sand for the rest of the year. My mammograms were thankfully always normal. I never had any lump or breast abnormality. What I did have was the feeling like it was coming. I just knew."

For Suzanne, the mammograms and waiting for the results were torture. "The nurse who always performed my mammogram was a sweet, sympathetic lady named Sandy, and I used to analyze every last word that came out of the poor woman's mouth," she says. "If she wished me good luck as I was leaving, I'd think, 'Why did she say that? What does she mean? Why didn't she just say "Have a good day" or "See you next year"? Will I need luck?' Then, from the day I'd have the mammogram to the day I got the letter saying everything was okay (which was often up to two weeks later). I'd drive myself crazy. I'd lie in bed at night, staring at the ceiling, thinking, 'This is it. This is the year I get cancer.' I'd be completely preoccupied with thoughts of death, imagining scenarios of going through chemo, losing my hair, my husband trying to raise our daughter on his own. I'd allow myself to go to those deep dark places—but just for those few weeks each year. It was the highest level of anxiety I've ever experienced.

"Then, after frantically running to the mailbox every day, I'd get the letter saying I was in the clear," Suzanne continues. "I'd immediately have an overwhelming sense of relief. I would thank God for letting me off the hook, and I'd start living in denial again until it was time for my mammogram the following year."

Though her story is sad, Suzanne acknowledges that at least she has no memories of watching her mother suffer. Mayde, on the other hand, does. "I was seventeen and had just started my freshman year of college when my mother had an aspiration of a cyst in her breast that had turned bloody," Mayde says. "She was admitted to the hospital for a surgical biopsy of the area where the cyst was found. It showed cancer, and she returned to the operating room for a radical mastectomy of that breast the very next day. The day after that, the doctors strongly suggested my mom have a mirror biopsy of her other breast, just to be safe. And when they found cancerous cells in the second breast, they decided to remove that one, too.

"I will never forget when I first saw my mom after her surgeries," Mayde continues. "My mother, Blossom, is the type of woman who is always well-coiffed and dressed impeccably. But there she was, lying in the hospital bed, hooked up to all these tubes. Some were pumping fluids into her body, while others were draining blood from her chest into these big plastic drums. My mom was comatose from the pain medication, and her chest was a horrifying sight—the doctors had removed not only her breasts but also her pectoral muscles and everything down to her ribs. She was flat as a board. I just stood there frozen, thinking, 'My mother isn't going to make it out of this hospital alive. How can I live without her? What's going to happen? Who's going to take care of me?' Even though I was pre-med and had volunteered at hospitals throughout high school, I just wasn't prepared to see my mother like that.

"My mom was in the hospital for two weeks and I sat with her every day," Mayde adds. "She'd slip in and out of consciousness, and when she awoke she'd usually vomit from all the narcotics. She couldn't eat or speak or even lift her arms because of the incisions from the surgery. My mother eventually did make it home, but she took a very long time to recover. She was in severe pain from nerve damage and developed lymphedema—because her lymph nodes were removed, the fluid in her body had nowhere to drain, causing one of her arms to swell up like a balloon. I took off from school for a few months so I could stay home and care for her.

"I was so damaged from seeing what my mother had endured," Mayde says. "But I never thought I'd ever have to do the same. I just hadn't yet made the connection that my mother's history could somehow affect me. Then, when I was twenty, I took my mother to see Dr. Roy Ashikari, the surgical oncologist who would wind up performing my mastectomy twenty-five years later. After he checked my mother, he turned to me, wagged his finger, and said in a stern voice, 'Be very careful all your life. Your mother had breast cancer. Always check yourself.' He made such an impression on me. It was like foreshadowing. That was the first time I realized, 'Hey, I'm at risk here.'"

While Suzanne's and Mayde's fear of breast cancer started with a bang, many women's worries begin more subtly. Take Lisa, for example. When she was a junior in high school, she felt a cluster of hard lumps in her left breast and her mother rushed her to a doctor to have them removed. "My mom's motto was, 'If it doesn't belong there, get it out,'" Lisa says. Lisa underwent general anesthesia and a surgery that left her with an unsightly three-inch scar across her breast. By the time she turned thirty, she had had three more biopsies of suspicious lumps and another one-inch scar above the previous one (the doctors were able to cut through previous incisions on some occasions). All turned out to be benign. "But each time, as I waited for the results, I'd think, 'Why is this happening?'" Lisa says. "At first, I'd have a 'Nothing can happen to me' frame of mind, but as I kept finding more lumps, I started having doubts." But this was just the beginning for Lisa. It wasn't until much later that her doubts turned into terror.

close calls

Whether waiting for the results from a biopsy or worrying about a suspicious mammogram or other indicator that breast cancer might strike, not knowing the prognosis is sometimes just as anxiety-provoking as hearing bad news, says Dr. Prigerson. "When there's a nonspecific dread that something horrible is going to happen, people tend to build up the likelihood of it in their minds and the fear takes on a life of its own," she says. "Once they know their results, they might still be terrified if the news is bad, but they can at least then start developing a game plan for dealing with it. Before that, they're just experiencing pure fear."

Amy knows what that waiting game is like all too well. She started getting mammograms when she was in her mid-twenties—fifteen years before the national recommendation—because of her family's history: Years after Amy's Grandma Ada died of breast cancer, her mother's younger sister fought the disease when she was only thirty-four. Then, after years of worrying about breast cancer, Amy's mom, Anne, got the diagnosis she always knew she'd get. She was fifty-three. "Luckily, my mom caught the breast cancer early, so she just had a lumpectomy and radiation," Amy says. "However, when it came back a few years later, she had a double mastectomy. Through it all, my mom was always strong. Her attitude was, 'I'm going to beat this.' And thankfully she did. I just couldn't imagine losing her—my mom was the center of my family, the glue that held us all together."

Amy's mammograms were uneventful until she was in her thirties. "One year, a few days after one of my mammograms, I was driving my three kids to see a movie when I got a call from my gynecologist's office," she says. "The doctor said, 'We saw something suspicious. You need to come back for additional pictures. Don't be alarmed.' I immediately thought, 'This is it. I have cancer.' Somehow, I pulled it together, got to the theater, bought tickets and popcorn, and shuttled my kids to their seats. I sat in that theater petrified, thinking, 'Here we go. My nightmare is coming true.' I felt numb and sick to my stomach.

"The next day, I went to an imaging center for an additional mammogram and an ultrasound," Amy continues. "After the tests, they left me to wait in this windowless room, wearing only a paper robe, feeling helpless. It could have been a minute or two, but it felt like forever. Then the radiologist came back in and said abruptly, 'Everything's okay. You can go home.' And that was it. I was elated, of course, but I also felt like a Mack truck had just hit me. I had a crushing headache and was so drained from the emotional roller coaster that I went home, collapsed into bed, and slept for hours.

"This mammogram was a huge wake-up call," Amy adds. "I always thought I'd get cancer someday, and now I was in my thirties and approaching the age my aunt was when she was diagnosed. It could be my turn soon."

Rori's big scare also came when a mammogram detected a lump when she was thirty-six. Cancer had ravaged most of her mother's family, one by one. First, her two great-aunts died of breast cancer; one uncle died of kidney cancer, another uncle of bladder cancer. Then Rori's mother, Lois, succumbed to ovarian cancer. A few years later, Rori's older sister, Lynne, battled the same disease.

So when Rori's doctors sent her in for a biopsy of the lump, needless to say she was very anxious. "I kept thinking about my mother, who I watched wither away," she says. "After many surgeries and months of chemo, she was skin and bones and feeling frightfully weak. Right before she died, she literally couldn't function. I don't know why—possibly the cancer had spread to her brain—but she was losing her memory and could barely scribble her name. She was so frail that I had to hold her in the shower and help her use the bathroom. She wasn't my mother anymore."

Rori also thought about her sister Lynne, who went into remission after eight rounds of chemo. "I never understood how someone so young could have cancer, and here I was with a lump and my history, thinking, 'I could be next,'" Rori says. "I prayed, 'Let me be cancer-free and I'll find a way to avoid being yet another link in the chain.'" After two biopsies (the doctors wanted to dig a little deeper the second time), she found out her lump was benign.

As for Mayde, after she witnessed her mother's horrific radical mastectomy when she was seventeen, her fears only grew in her twenties and thirties as she graduated from medical school, started her podiatry practice, and eventually married Jonathan, who is a radiologist. "Being completely immersed in the world of medicine, I became so aware of my risk that it was always at the forefront of my mind," Mayde says. She also became particularly frightened when she kept finding suspicious cysts. "I really started getting nervous because my mom always went for cyst aspirations," she says. "I thought, 'Uh-oh, I'm following in her footsteps.'" Mayde had to have three of her cysts biopsied; each time, little pieces of one of her breasts were removed. "I felt like I was being chipped away," she says.

Then, one of Mayde's biggest scares came two days after she gave birth to her first child, Phoebe. "I was lying in the hospital bed trying to nurse, but my daughter was having trouble latching on," she recalls. "The nurses brought in a breast pump and, when I started pumping, the fluid that came out of the left breast was tinged with blood. My husband and the nurses looked puzzled and somewhat panicked. A breast surgeon came in and took a sample of the fluid. I wasn't allowed to nurse on that side, and I 'pumped and dumped' while I waited for the results. I remember gazing at my precious newborn and thinking, 'I can't believe this is happening during the happiest time of my life.'"

A few days later, the tests came back inconclusive, and since there was no more blood in the milk the surgeon told Mayde they'd just take the "wait-and-see" approach. "I was so overjoyed with my baby that I tried to focus on her and nothing else," Mayde says. "But I couldn't help thinking, 'Something is brewing.'" It would turn out she was right.

the last straw

Fear is a living, breathing thing. The more it's nourished, the stronger it gets. As it grows, it becomes so powerful that it can actually consume a person completely. And that's exactly the point when these five women each realized they had had enough.

Lisa, for example, always thought that having lumps biopsied and being left with scars was just something she had to deal with. But then her mother was diagnosed with breast cancer when Lisa was twenty-nine. "Once my mother got cancer, I woke up and realized, 'I can get this, too.' After that, every time I'd find a lump, I'd panic.

I had terrible anxiety and would experience tightness in my chest. I started constantly doing breast exams in the shower and was always thinking, 'Mom's sick, and I'm going to turn out just like her.'"

Lisa and her mom, Arlene, were best friends. "We did everything together—shopping at flea markets, playing backgammon, taking my kids to Gymboree," Lisa says. "We had the same thick New York accent and even looked alike, though her curls were red and mine are dark brown. Then one day my mom found a lump and immediately went to the doctor to get it checked. I'll never forget when she called me and said the words no one ever wants to hear: 'I have cancer.' I was driving and I started crying so hard I had to pull over. Those few words shattered my world."

Arlene had a lumpectomy, followed by chemo and radiation. "That's when I really became frightened because my mom began to look ill," says Lisa. "She was exhausted and often nauseous, and she shaved off all her beautiful curls because she didn't want to deal with losing them bit by bit. Her wigs were hot and itchy, so she'd usually just wear a bandana. People would sometimes stare at her, and I'd be like a mother hen, trying to distract her so she didn't notice. I was so overwhelmed with seeing my mother suffer that after dinner with my family, I'd lock myself in my home office and just weep. I even left my demanding corporate marketing job because, in part, I wanted to be around to help my mother in any way that I could. To me, time with her was too precious."

Arlene's treatment seemed to work, but five years later the breast cancer metastasized to her bones and she had to start chemo and radiation all over again. This time, she was living with a chronic illness, and the doctors were focused on giving her the best quality of life possible and preventing the cancer from spreading further. Every few months, they'd whip up a different cocktail of medication. When that stopped working, they'd try another.

Then, while on a family vacation in New York two years later, Lisa received a call from her brother. He said that their mom had taken a turn for the worse.

"What are you talking about?" Lisa asked.

"Lisa, it's really bad," her brother said. "You have to come home."

"What do you mean?" she said. "Can I talk to Mom?"

"No. She can't talk. You have to get home. I think this is the end."

"I couldn't believe it," Lisa says. "My mom had just left me a message on my cell phone the day before asking about my trip and telling me how much she missed me. I was in shock but somehow composed myself, got on a flight back to Florida the next morning, and raced from the airport directly to the hospital.

"When I reached the ICU, all I kept thinking was, it can't be *that* bad," she continues. "Well, it was. The cancer was in my mom's liver, and overnight she had become unconscious, filling with fluid, and turning bright yellow. I screamed when I saw her. The woman lying in that bed didn't look anything like my mother. That's when I became hysterical. I whispered in her ear, 'Mom, I wish I could help you!' My brother told me that Mom was completely out of it because she was on so much morphine, but she suddenly squeezed my hand really hard. I felt she was trying to tell me that she knew I was there. I just cried, held her hand, and told her I loved her. She died within minutes. I watched the monitor as her heart rate began to slow. It was a countdown to death. In my heart, I knew she was ready to go, but I wasn't ready to let her go. I just stood there and stared at my mother, dead. The disease finally beat us. No more Mom. No more Grandma Arlene. That was the moment when my life would never be the same again."

The following year, while Lisa was still deeply mourning her mother, she became more vigilant than ever about screening. She went for an ultrasound, and this time the test showed two lumps in her right breast—two lumps that Lisa had never felt herself. "That really scared me," she says. "I had found all my previous lumps, but never noticed these. What if they were the ones that turned out to be cancerous?" And though they weren't, Lisa says that she had had it. "My mother had just died, and I was so sick of this disease. I was done dealing with breast cancer."

For Suzanne, she always had the threat of breast cancer looming over her, particularly since her mother died from it when Suzanne was only four. However, her last straw was mistakenly being told she had the disease. At the time, she was contemplating undergoing genetic testing and was meeting with an oncologist who asked her to bring along her recent mammogram. That mammogram, it turned out, had a slight change from the previous year and Suzanne was going to get an MRI the very next day to make sure that everything was okay.

"When I first met with the oncologist, she took my mammogram and put it up on a light board in her office's reception area," Suzanne says. "She studied it for what seemed like hours and then began pacing back and forth."

"There's something wrong, isn't there?" Suzanne asked.

The oncologist sat down next to her and took her hand. "I see it," she said, her eyes staring directly into Suzanne's. "I see the spot they are talking about. This is very, very serious. You need to have a biopsy immediately."

The whole office froze. The patients within earshot became absolutely silent. Suzanne felt like the room was closing in on her. Everything went blank and she could feel the blood draining out of her face. There was an eerie white noise in her head, like something out of an Alfred Hitchcock movie.

"You see cancer?" she asked.

The doctor nodded.

"Are you sure?"

"Well, the only thing that is one hundred percent sure is a biopsy, so I am having my secretary call the best surgeon we know and we'll see how soon you can get in," she responded.

At this point Suzanne wasn't really sure what the doctor was talking about. Since the mammogram only showed a cloudy area, she was thinking, "There is no lump. There's nothing to biopsy." But Suzanne took her word for it and said, "You're an oncologist. This is your field. You *know* what cancer looks like."

The doctor nodded.

"Is it invasive?" Suzanne asked.

She nodded again and said, "Invasive ductal carcinoma."

Suzanne thought, "Here we go. I'm just like my mom. People don't survive cancer in my family, so why should I?" Again, she was picturing herself going for chemo treatments, her daughter growing up without her just like she grew up without her mom. She couldn't foresee one step at a time. She jumped right to: "I'm dead."

Suzanne immediately called Mayde, who had become a mentor of sorts since she was the person who had encouraged Suzanne to confront her risk in the first place. The next day, Suzanne headed to Mayde's husband's radiology practice for her MRI. Mayde went with her for moral support and to make sure everything ran smoothly. "As soon as the test was done, Mayde ran to the room where the breast imaging specialist was evaluating my results," Suzanne recalls. "I was in a chair at the other end of the hall, and when I saw her lean out of the radiologist's room and give me a thumbs-up, I started sobbing. I almost collapsed and needed my husband, Pascal, to hold me up. I had been so convinced I had breast cancer that the relief was overwhelming. But I also knew the relief would be short-lived. I thought, 'Today I'm fine. But what about tomorrow?' I just couldn't take this waiting game anymore."

While Lisa and Suzanne can pinpoint the exact incidents that put them over the edge, Amy cannot. "It was as though all signs were pointing to breast cancer," she says. "First, there was my family history and that horrible mammogram scare, but one day my best friend from college, a mom of two young children, called to tell me she had breast cancer. That scared me beyond belief. How could this happen to her? It was supposed to be me.

"Then a mom at my kids' school was going through chemo," Amy continues. "The disease was just everywhere. And every time I heard about someone who got cancer, I thought, 'That could be me.' I then had a second mammogram scare and began looking at everyone as a statistic. I'd be on the tennis court and I'd think, 'Okay, if one in eight women get breast cancer in their lifetime and there are sixteen girls on my team, that means two of us will likely get breast cancer. I'll be one of them. I wonder who the other will be?' I knew this was not a way to live."

What made matters worse was the fact that Amy couldn't really discuss her fears with too many people. From the time her mom was diagnosed with breast cancer, her parents and siblings always had the attitude of "What happens in the family stays in the family." Amy couldn't tell anyone but her closest friends what her mom was going through. When she went to a hospital in Miami for her mother's mastectomy, for example, she didn't even tell anyone where she was. Then, years later, when dealing with her own suspicious mammograms, Amy barely talked about it. "I had the same kind of attitude as my mom—I'll deal with this and move on," she says. However tormented she might be, dealing with cancer—even just the possibility of it—was a private matter.

one more factor

For each of these five women, fear originated from a different source and manifested itself in unique ways. But the one commonality that helped push each of them over the edge was the fact that they were all moms.

"When you have kids, life in general is just scarier because, as the saying goes, there's a little piece of your heart out there in the world," says Rori, a mom of two boys and a girl. "I feel such a strong need to protect my kids, and I'm determined to leave them at a ripe old age. Of course, I could get hit by a car tomorrow, but there's no way I was going to let cancer get me."

Rori explains that her conviction comes from dealing with her mother's death when she was thirty. "My mom was my life," she says. "I lost my father to kidney failure when I was fourteen, so she was all I had. I loved her more than anything. Just like me, my mom was a happy-go-lucky free spirit who taught me about finding the best in people. She was adventurous and glamorous, and she embraced every aspect of life—from traveling and fashion to art, food, and music. Even when I was an adult, she made every day together so exciting. I felt so empty when I lost her to ovarian cancer, and my life has never been the same since. It breaks my heart just thinking of my kids' ever experiencing the same pain."

Lisa agrees. "My mom and I used to talk on the phone at least two or three times every day, and I still often reach for the phone to call her, even years after her death. I'm so devastated not having my mother with me, and I'm not willing to let my three kids go through what I've been through. They lost their grandmother. That's enough."

"It's a matter of responsibility," Mayde adds. "When I was single and didn't have anyone depending on me, the threat of breast cancer was scary. But once I had my son and daughter, the fear hit a whole new level. I wasn't just afraid for myself anymore. I was afraid for them."

Like many moms, Amy thinks of logistics. "With three kids, I just don't have time to get sick and deal with having breast cancer," she says. "I have to keep up with them."

As for Suzanne, she never really understood what it meant not to have a mom until she became one herself. "After I adopted my daughter, Nina (named after my mom), I realized how profound my loss was," she says. "I didn't have that person who loves you unconditionally and knows every little idiosyncratic thing about you. For instance, I know that the only kind of orange juice Nina will drink is pulp-free Tropicana in a plastic cup with a straw, and that she wears shoes a size too big because she doesn't like feeling them on her feet. Sure, I had some motherly influences in my life. When I was a kid my dance teacher, Miss Bonnii, would do my hair and makeup before my recitals, while all the other girls in my class had their moms fussing over them. But when I got married, no one helped me pick out my dress or plan my wedding. No one showed me how to change a diaper or swaddle a baby when Nina was an infant. If I could help it, there was no way I'd let my daughter miss out on all the things I missed by not having my mother around. I decided I'd do whatever I could to make sure I was there for her."

what's my risk?

While it's one thing to think you might have an elevated risk for breast cancer, to *know* it is an entirely different ball game. And deciding to face that truth, one that can bring with it major health implications and emotional turmoil, is a very personal decision. Like many women, Amy always figured she had a high risk, but she never wanted to deal with it. "I was busy raising my children, living my life, and I just wasn't ready," she says. "But then I went through that whole experience where there was something suspicious on my mammogram and I had to go back for an ultrasound. That's when I changed my tune. I was so freaked out because, even though the ultrasound eventually showed that I was okay, I knew the next time I might not be. I had three kids and was not getting any younger. It was time for me to know what kind of risk I was contending with."

We are all at risk for breast cancer to some degree (even men aren't immune). Of course, not all risk is created equal. For instance, the average woman has a one-in-eight chance of developing breast cancer during her lifetime. A person with previous breast biopsies and a family history, as Lisa had, might have around 30 percent odds. But for someone like Suzanne, who shares the genetic mutation that likely attributed to the deaths of most of her family, a woman's chances can be as high as a staggering 87 percent.

Finding out your risk for breast cancer can be upsetting and, at times, overwhelming, but it also can be the first step toward defying your fate. "By really understanding a woman's individual risk, it's possible to tailor her screening prevention methods," says Rebecca Sutphen, M.D., a leading risk assessment expert and recent director of clinical genetics at Moffitt Cancer Center in Tampa. "Otherwise, everyone would have the same plan, which logically shouldn't be the case." What Dr. Sutphen is referring to is "personalized medicine," which is when doctors use a patient's genetic and clinical information as well as family history to come up with a medication, therapy, or preventative measure appropriate for that person at that time. For instance, while the average woman might just need a yearly mammogram, someone with a higher risk might want to consider adding breast MRI to her surveillance. Without knowing a person's specific risk, screening and prevention simply become one-size-fits-all.

the risk factors

When it comes to breast cancer, a risk factor is anything that makes a person more susceptible than other people to getting the disease. According to the American Cancer Society, one or more of the genetic or environmental risks listed below can raise your odds of getting breast cancer—in some cases, slightly; in others, dramatically.

But before you become overwhelmed by all the statistics, know that these factors affect everyone differently—just because, say, drinking alcohol might increase someone else's risk for developing breast cancer, that doesn't mean it will for you. In fact, having any or all of these factors doesn't guarantee you'll get cancer, just as not having any of them doesn't mean that a person will not get the disease. Also, don't start adding or subtracting your risk based on these data—it doesn't work that way. You can't add an increase in risk due to taking birth control pills to an increase linked to having gotten your period early. If Mayde did that, for instance, her risk would have been well over 100 percent—she can check "yes" next to most of the factors listed below.

The key is to simply know which of the following factors pertain to you so you can talk to your doctor about *your* odds of getting breast cancer.

GENDER

Being a woman is the biggest risk factor for developing breast cancer, primarily because the female hormones estrogen and progesterone continually stimulate breast cell growth. Men can develop breast cancer, too, but women are approximately one hundred times more likely to get the disease.

AGE

The older a woman is, the greater her risk of developing breast cancer. Essentially, the longer a person is alive, the more time her breast cells have to go through the abnormal changes that cause cancer. In fact, 87.5 percent of all breast cancer diagnoses are among women over the age of forty-five; around 65 percent are over the age of fifty-five.

GENETIC LINK

Experts generally consider 5 percent to 10 percent of breast cancer cases to be hereditary, which means a person has inherited a mutated gene that directly increases the odds of getting the disease. Genes are instruction manuals that tell our bodies how to operate, and we all have two copies of each of them—one from our mothers and one from our fathers. Usually a mutation (or change) in a gene is harmless. But a mutation in certain genes can greatly impact a woman's risk of getting breast cancer.

Here are the ones we know of so far:

- **Breast cancer genes, known as BRCA1 and BRCA2** (pronounced brak-uh): We're all born with two tumor suppressor genes, called BRCA1 and BRCA2, which are meant to control the growth of cells in the breasts and ovaries. When these genes are not functioning properly, which is the case in from one in three hundred to one in eight hundred people, such cells can grow and reproduce too rapidly, resulting in cancer. If a woman inherits a dysfunctional copy of either gene from her mother or father, her risk for developing breast and ovarian cancer compounds significantly. Some studies estimate up to an 87 percent lifetime risk for breast cancer and up to a 44 percent lifetime risk for ovarian cancer. (Note: These estimates indicate the high end of what a woman's odds will be. Some people with mutations will have lower odds, but because there is not yet a way for experts to indicate a woman's *exact* risk, they can only offer the vague "up to" an 87 percent and 44 percent risk. However, researchers predict that someday soon they'll be able to give women a more precise risk assessment.) BRCA mutations also may slightly increase a woman's risk of other cancers, such as melanoma and pancreatic cancer. They raise the risk for breast and prostate cancer among men, and in women who have already battled breast cancer, a second occurrence. Among carriers, cancer tends to strike at a younger age than in the general population. Last, it's important to note that genes cannot skip a generation. For instance, if your paternal grandfather has the BRCA2 gene mutation but your father does not, you can't inherit it from that side of the family. However, if you have a mutation, you have a 50 percent chance of passing it on to each of your kids.

- **PTEN gene:** Mutations in this tumor suppressor gene cause most cases of Cowden syndrome, a rare disorder that leads to an increased risk of certain diseases, such as breast, uterine, and thyroid cancers. Other signs and symptoms include noncancerous growths, thyroid changes, lipomas (benign fatty tumors under the skin), uterine fibroids, fibrocystic breast disease, mental disability, and an enlarged head size. Specifically, having this syndrome puts women at a 25 to 50 percent risk for developing breast cancer during their lifetime. However, the PTEN genetic mutation which causes it is much less common than BRCA mutations.

- **p53 gene:** Also a tumor suppressor gene, mutations in p53 can cause Li-Fraumeni syndrome, characterized by cancers such as breast cancer, leukemia, brain tumors, bone cancer, and soft tissue sarcoma. Typically, multiple tumors will appear in the same person or within the same family, often at young ages. People with this rare mutation have up to a 50 percent risk of the associated cancers by age fifty.

- **ATM, CHEK2 genes:** Inherited variants of these genes and others like them can raise a person's risk of getting breast cancer—some experts say they double it—though not nearly as high as the genetic mutations mentioned above.

- **Future genes:** Some experts predict that in the next five years as many as one hundred genetic mutations or alterations linked to breast cancer will be discovered, and that up to 50 percent of all breast cancer cases will carry a hereditary component.

"We say BRCA and a few other mutations cause 5 to 10 percent of all breast cancers, but we are really only referring to the ones that cause a major predisposition," explains Dr. Sutphen. "We don't know all the genes that give women double or triple the average risk. It may turn out many more people have a genetic tendency toward breast cancer." See Chapter 14 for more information about the future of genetics.

PERSONAL HISTORY OF BREAST CANCER

A woman who has developed cancer in one breast has up to four times an increased risk of cancer in the other breast or in a different part of the same breast. This is not considered a recurrence of the initial cancer; it is a brand-new cancer. It's important to note that a growing number of women who have been diagnosed with breast cancer might try to prevent a second occurrence by having both breasts removed (even the healthy one). While these women are still considered survivors, their actions are also similar to those of some previvors.

FAMILY HISTORY OF BREAST CANCER

Breast cancer risk is greater among women whose blood relatives have had the disease, particularly if they were diagnosed before menopause. Having one first-degree relative (mother, sister, or daughter) with breast cancer doubles a woman's risk. Each additional relative increases the odds. For instance, one recent study found that BRCA-negative women who have two or more relatives diagnosed with breast cancer before fifty or three or more relatives diagnosed at any age have a fourfold increased risk of developing the disease themselves. A history of breast cancer in a close male relative also significantly increases a woman's risk.

RACE AND ETHNICITY

White women have higher odds of developing breast cancer than African-American women. However, African-American women are more likely to die from breast cancer, somewhat because they are more prone to developing an aggressive form of the disease. Asian, Hispanic, and Native American women have a lower risk of both getting breast cancer and dying from it. Although BRCA mutations can occur in any racial or ethnic group, they are more common among certain populations. For instance, Jewish people of Ashkenazi (Eastern Europe) descent have a one in forty chance of having a BRCA mutation, more than ten times the general population's odds.

ABNORMAL BREAST BIOPSY RESULTS

Some types of benign breast conditions seem to raise breast cancer risk; others don't. Those that are proliferative (which means that the cells are rapidly multiplying) can increase risk. Those that aren't, like cysts, usually do not. And of the proliferative conditions, those with atypia (which means an abnormality appears in the cell) seem to raise risk up to five times higher than normal, such as atypical ductal hyperplasia (ADH) and atypical lobular hyperplasia (ALH). Women with LCIS (lobular carcinoma in situ) have ten times the risk of developing invasive cancer within their lifetime, according to the Mayo Clinic. Other conditions that are proliferative but don't have atypia also raise risk, but only one and a half to two times higher than normal.

RADIATION EXPOSURE

Women who have had radiation therapy to the chest area for Hodgkin's lymphoma, non-Hodgkin's lymphoma, or other cancers have much higher odds of developing breast cancer, particularly if they were treated during adolescence. The higher the dose of radiation and the earlier the treatment, the greater the risk.

BREAST DENSITY

Women with dense breasts, meaning that they have a greater proportion of breast tissue to fat as seen on their mammogram, are more likely to develop breast cancer than those women with lower-density breasts. There's also a risk that a woman with dense breasts who does get cancer will be diagnosed later because fat tissue appears black on a mammogram, while breast tissue and tumors both appear white. For that reason, spotting a tumor in dense breast tissue can be difficult, like "trying to find a white speck in a snowstorm," says Debbie Saslow, Ph.D., director of breast and gynecologic cancers at the American Cancer Society.

HORMONE-RELATED INFLUENCES

According to the National Cancer Institute, prolonged exposure to estrogen may increase a woman's risk of breast cancer. Estrogen does not cause cancer, but it does stimulate cells in our bodies to duplicate and grow. This is a normal process. At the same time, cells are constantly mutating within our bodies. Mutated cells are not cancer and, in most cases, will die off. However, when estrogen binds to breast cells that already have a genetic error, the theory is that it can accelerate the growth of cancer. Experts believe that the more estrogen we have in our bodies, the more likely this will happen. Factors that influence estrogen levels include:

- **Menstrual periods**
  Women who get their periods at an early age (before age twelve) or those who go through menopause at a late age (after

age fifty-five) have slightly greater odds of getting breast cancer. Since estrogen levels are highest when a woman is menstruating, the thought is that the more lifetime periods a woman has, the more estrogen her body is exposed to through the years.

- **Number of births**

  The relationship between pregnancy and breast cancer is a complicated one. On the one hand, women who have never given birth to children or who had their first child after age thirty have a somewhat higher chance of developing breast cancer. Pregnancy not only decreases the number of lifetime menstrual cycles, but experts believe it also somehow changes breast tissue, making it less likely to become cancerous in the long run. The earlier a woman has children, the sooner she'll gain this beneficial effect. And the more children she has, the greater the protection. However, according to the National Cancer Institute, a woman's breast cancer risk is temporarily increased within the few years after she gives birth.

- **Birth control pills**

  Some research shows that women on oral contraceptives have a greater risk of breast cancer than women who have never taken them. However, a woman's risk seems to return to normal within ten years after she stops usage. Keep in mind that birth control pills have also been shown to have many health benefits, such as lowering a woman's odds of developing ovarian and endometrial cancers. Talk to your doctor about whether or not they're right for you.

- **Hormone replacement therapy**

  Hormone replacement therapy (HRT) helps relieve symptoms of menopause and prevent osteoporosis. Yet in the most comprehensive study on the topic to date, the Women's Health Initiative found that long-term use of combined estrogen plus progestin therapy increases a woman's risk of breast cancer by 24 percent.

This risk seems to diminish within three years after discontinuing use. The study also found that women who had hysterectomies and take estrogen-only HRT had no increased risk, though other research shows that prolonged use of it does. The Food and Drug Administration and other health agencies and organizations recommend that women who take any form of HRT choose the lowest dose that helps for the shortest time possible.

- **Breast-feeding**
  Breast-feeding appears to lower breast cancer risk, particularly if it is continued for one and a half to two years. The longer the better. Again, estrogen is possibly the key factor—since a woman's menstrual cycle typically stops while breast-feeding, she'll decrease her breasts' lifetime exposure to the hormone.

BEING OVERWEIGHT

Gaining weight as an adult increases postmenopausal breast cancer risk. The reason why such effects occur later in life is that before menopause, most of a woman's estrogen is produced by her ovaries. However, after menopause, the ovaries stop making estrogen, and fat tissue becomes the primary source of the hormone. The more fat in a woman's body, the greater her estrogen levels, which, in turn, increase the odds of developing breast cancer. In fact, a study by the American Cancer Society found that women who gained twenty-one to thirty pounds since age eighteen were 40 percent more likely to develop breast cancer than women who had not gained more than five pounds. Women who gained seventy pounds doubled their risk.

PHYSICAL ACTIVITY

More studies are starting to show that exercise reduces breast cancer risk, possibly because it lowers women's estrogen levels and acts indirectly to help with weight control. For instance, one study from the Women's Health Initiative found that postmenopausal women who walked about 1¼ to 2½ hours per week had 18 percent less risk than women who were inactive. The American Cancer Society recommends that women exercise for forty-five to sixty minutes five to seven days a week.

LOW-FAT DIET

Data are not yet clear on whether or not eating low-fat foods can decrease a woman's risk of breast cancer. Of course, eating a diet high in fat can lead to a higher calorie consumption, cause weight gain, and, indirectly, lead to an increased risk. In general, the American Cancer Society advises eating five or more servings of vegetables and fruits each day, choosing whole grains over processed grains, and limiting consumption of processed and red meats.

ALCOHOL

Drinking more than one alcoholic drink a day increases a woman's odds of developing breast cancer. The more alcohol consumed, the greater the risk, regardless whether your beverage of choice is beer, liquor, or wine. Compared with nondrinkers, women who drink one alcoholic beverage a day have a very slight increase in risk. Those who have two to five drinks daily have approximately 1½ times the risk. Some experts hypothesize that this occurs because alcohol can raise a woman's estrogen levels.

understanding risk

You might know which factors put you at a higher risk for developing breast cancer. But by how much? That's where it gets a little tricky. If you're going to be making decisions based on your perceived risk, it's important to have a good understanding of what the numbers mean. A quick tutorial:

> **Absolute risk** is the odds a person will develop breast cancer over a specific time period. For example, you can determine your odds in the next year, the next five years, or throughout your lifetime. So when you hear the well-known statistic that one in eight women will develop breast cancer during their lifetime, that's an absolute risk.
>
> **Relative risk** shows the relationship between a risk factor and breast cancer by comparing a group of people who have that particular risk with people who don't.

For instance, say a particular group of women has a 20 percent lifetime chance of getting breast cancer. That 20 percent is those women's absolute risk. If they could each take a pill and reduce that risk from 20 percent to 10 percent, the absolute improvement is 10 percent, while the relative reduction is 50 percent. Essentially, the absolute risk gives you a more honest number, but the risk you typically hear about in the media is relative. When you do hear reports of a particular lifestyle change that can lower your risk of breast cancer by 25 percent, you need to know your original risk. If it was high, say 60 percent, then 25 percent of 60 is 15 percent, which would be a significant reduction. But if your risk were only 10 percent to begin with, decreasing it by 25 percent would just equal 2½ percent.

first steps

Chances are you already have a hunch that you or someone you know has a higher than average risk for developing breast cancer. But how do you even begin to tackle your odds? Often, the first line of defense lies with your gynecologist or family doctor. The American College of Obstetricians and Gynecologists guidelines state that most clinicians are "capable of basic genetic risk identification and counseling" and "able to elicit an accurate history and document risk factors that might increase the patient's risk of developing breast cancer." However, doctors often don't bring up such issues, not out of negligence but because they just don't have the time or the training in genetics to discuss them.

In other words, it's crucial to take charge of your own health. "The whole 'Don't ask, don't tell' concept just doesn't apply here," says David Fishman, M.D., director of gynecologic oncology research and the Cancer Detection and Screening Program at Mount Sinai School of Medicine in New York. Even if your doctor doesn't bring it up, tell him or her about any cancers in your family, risk factors you might personally have, and other important details you think he or she should know. "At that point, your doctor should be able to either advise you or, if he or she believes your medical needs lie outside their area of expertise, refer you to an expert who can help," says Dr. Fishman.

Suzanne knows all too well the importance of being your own advocate. Though her history on her mother's side was astounding— her mother, Nina, died young from breast cancer, her grandfather from lung cancer, her grandmother from what they now think was ovarian cancer, and two of her mother's siblings from lung cancer and leukemia (a third sibling is a breast cancer survivor)—no doctor ever suggested that Suzanne go for genetic counseling or testing. In fact, when researchers first discovered the BRCA1 gene in 1994, Suzanne asked her primary care physician about it. His response was, "Don't get tested. You'll never get health insurance again." (Years later, she learned this wasn't true.) "Nobody said to me, 'You have these red flags, you need to have further testing,'" Suzanne says. "I didn't realize how much I was at risk or what measures I should be taking until the day I first struck up a conversation with Mayde, whose daughter was in a dance class I was teaching. When Mayde found out my mom had died of breast cancer, *she* was the one who pushed me to get an MRI. She suggested I consider getting genetic testing. She did more to inform me in that one-hour conversation than did so many visits with my doctor. Thanks to her encouragement, I eventually started taking steps to protect myself."

Bottom line: Talk to your family physician or gynecologist about your risk, but always trust your instincts. Even if your doctor tells you that you have nothing to worry about, at least get a second opinion (ideally from a genetics expert) if you're still in doubt.

EVALUATING GENERAL RISK ASSESSMENT MODELS

Online assessment methods exist to help experts determine your risk for breast cancer and your risk for having a BRCA mutation. However, each of these methods has limitations and should only be used to get a ballpark idea of where your risk might lie. Keep in mind that your risk estimate might vary based on which tool you use.

SOME OF THE MOST COMMON ASSESSMENT MODELS:

Gail Model: This popular tool helps determine a woman's risk for getting breast cancer. However, the method is only useful for the average woman *without* an extensive family history of cancer. (For instance, the model doesn't take into account the ages family members were diagnosed, second-degree relatives with the disease, or any history of cancer on the father's side.) Though the Gail Model is accessible via the National Cancer Institute website (www.cancer.gov/bcrisktool), a woman should still contact a genetics expert to review her family history and risk for breast cancer.

Claus Model: This model also helps determine breast cancer risk, and unlike the Gail Model, it takes both maternal and paternal family history into consideration. However, the Claus Model is limited in that it doesn't take into account any risk factors except family history.

BRCAPRO: This model assesses a person's chance of having a BRCA1 or BRCA2 mutation. However, it doesn't include hormonal factors such as age of first period or a woman's personal history of breast biopsies, atypia, and other abnormal findings.

Other online methods: There are various tools and calculators online that attempt to determine a woman's risk. Again, remember that none of these tools can replace a full evaluation by a professional who understands these models' limitations and can better explain their findings. Suzanne, for instance, used an online BRCA risk calculator to help determine if she was at risk for having a genetic mutation. According to the calculator, her risk was surprisingly only 4.5 percent. Her genetic counselor suggested she might as well undergo genetic testing anyway just to completely rule out the possibility that she had a BRCA mutation. Suzanne followed her advice, and a few days later, headed off to St. Barts for a vacation with friends. "I really thought I didn't have to worry and was off lying on the beach, relaxing without a care in the world," Suzanne recalls. "But, sure enough, when I returned, I found out that I had tested positive for BRCA2. I personally never would have relied on that one online evaluation to accurately assess my risk, but it's scary to think how wrong it was."

is genetic counseling for you?

It might be overwhelming to confront your risk, but you don't have to do so alone. A genetic counselor or any medical expert specifically trained in genetics can be incredibly helpful while you're learning about your odds of getting breast cancer. "Genetics is a complicated, constantly evolving field, and it can be very difficult for a person to get a clear understanding of their risk unless they have input from a specialist in that area," says Sue Friedman, founder and director of FORCE, a national support network for women with a high risk for breast and ovarian cancer. Board-certified genetics experts can provide you with accurate, up-to-date information about your risk, help you with the psychological repercussions of knowing it, and explain all of your options so you can make an informed decision regarding what, if anything, to do about it. The danger of making such decisions "in a vacuum," as Friedman puts it, is that women may make potentially life-altering choices based on false information or data they don't comprehend. That's why it is absolutely vital that you seek the help of an expert when confronting your risk.

Rori understands the importance of such counseling. Though she didn't rush to get genetic counseling when her mother was diagnosed with ovarian cancer (a warning sign that Rori might be at risk for both ovarian and breast cancer), she knew she had no choice when her sister was diagnosed with the same disease. "At that point, I had such an intense feeling something hereditary was going on in my family, I decided I needed some answers," Rori says. "Sure, I was scared to take that next step, but seeking help was one of the best decisions I ever made. My counselor, Talia, really explained the pros and cons of genetic testing and, afterward, helped me understand and deal with my positive results." Of course, not everyone who goes for counseling winds up getting genetic testing. But the key is to at least educate yourself. Nothing can happen to you by talking to someone and becoming informed.

According to the National Comprehensive Cancer Network, here are some signs that might make you want to consider genetic counseling:

- You or a close family member under the age of fifty has been diagnosed with breast cancer.
- There are two or more cases of breast cancer in your family.
- There's any ovarian cancer in your family (this includes fallopian tube and primary peritoneal cancer).
- There's male breast cancer in your family.
- You or a close family member has had two separately diagnosed breast cancers or both breast and ovarian cancer.
- There's breast cancer and any other kind of cancer in your family (brain tumors, pancreatic cancer, thyroid cancer, etc.).
- A member of your family has a known BRCA mutation (or other hereditary breast cancer syndrome).
- You're among a population that has a higher risk for having the BRCA gene mutation (e.g., Ashkenazi Jews).

HOW TO FIND A GENETICS EXPERT

If you choose to seek professional help, here are some sites that can help you locate a board-certified genetics expert in your area:

National Society of Genetic Counselors
(www.nsgc.org/resourcelink.cfm)
    Allows you to search for counselors by location, name, institution, or areas of practice or specialization.

National Cancer Institute (www.cancer.gov)

Check out the Cancer Genetics Services Directory, which allows you to search for genetics experts by name, location, or specialty.

FORCE (www.facingourrisk.org)

Provides referrals via a hotline number (866-288-RISK) and e-mail (info@facingourrisk.org).

Informed Medical Decisions (www.informeddna.com or toll-free 1-800-975-4819)

Provides counseling over the phone with board-certified genetics experts. Most major health insurers will at least partially reimburse for this service, which is available by appointment (nights and weekends, too).

WHAT TO EXPECT

A genetic counseling session, which an increasing number of insurance companies are beginning to cover, usually involves an in-depth discussion about a woman's medical history as well as that of her family. The expert will want to know such history going back as far as possible. Improve your odds of getting an accurate risk assessment by bringing the following information to your appointment:

- Your medical records, including any notes or pathology reports regarding previous biopsies.
- The ages of any family members who were diagnosed with cancer and the main site of the cancers (e.g., "began in the breast and spread to the lungs").
- Original pathology reports of such diagnoses if you have them.
- The ages of living family members and the causes of and ages at death of those who have passed away.

- Any family health details you think might be worth mentioning.

Usually, a genetics expert will begin by drawing your family tree by using the information you provide. Based on that diagram and possibly one of the risk assessment tools such as the Gail Model, the counselor will then talk about the odds that you have hereditary breast cancer in your family. If it seems like you do, she will likely offer genetic testing and will discuss its benefits, risks, and limitations as well as possible financial and insurance implications. She might also discuss the psychological impact that testing can have on you and your family. If you determine that testing is not appropriate, the expert can then discuss what your next step might be. If you do get tested, you'll meet with the genetic counselor again and often an oncologist or other medical expert once your results come back. Regardless of the outcome of the test, they can walk you through the surveillance and preventative options available to you. Last, the counselor will usually send you or your referring physician a report summarizing everything discussed in your meeting.

Lisa's experience is somewhat typical. She always had a history of lumps and multiple biopsies, but when her mother, Arlene, was diagnosed with breast cancer she wanted to discuss her options with a genetics expert. Through a referral from her gynecologist, Lisa made an appointment with Dr. Louise Morrell, an oncologist specifically trained in genetics. "When I first entered Dr. Morrell's office, I was nervous, but she smiled and offered me a seat," Lisa recalls. "She then told me she was going to take my complete medical history, and said, 'Go relative by relative as far back as you can and see what you can remember.' I told her about my mom's recent diagnosis of breast cancer, my uncle's prostate cancer, and my grandfather's breast cancer, which I later found out is a major red flag. As I spoke, she started drawing a diagram, linking each of my family members together. When we were finished, I was shocked. Cancer was all the way up the chain. It's like she was putting a puzzle together, and when all the pieces were in place it was so obvious that there must be some sort of genetic link to cancer in my family. I just never saw it before. That first meeting with Dr. Morrell was upsetting but very enlightening. I felt like I was finally starting to have a clue of what kind of risk I was really dealing with."

to test or not to test

When a woman thinks she has a high risk for breast cancer, often one of her biggest concerns is that she carries a BRCA mutation (or, in some cases, other genetic mutations). But even if all signs indicate that such a hereditary factor is present, that doesn't mean genetic testing is for everyone. Of course, in some instances it is absolutely the right decision. But in others, testing might not be medically indicated or a woman might not be ready to deal with the consequences of finding out she's positive. Most experts say that women should only consider testing if the results will be useful. In other words, if the outcome won't change how you manage your risk and you don't have any relatives who can benefit from the information, genetic testing might not be right for you.

Someone who has already been diagnosed with breast cancer might also want to test for several reasons. Having a BRCA mutation would let that person know she's at an increased risk for ovarian cancer and, as new research strongly suggests, a second breast cancer. Such a result would also indicate implications for her family's cancer risk as well.

While a genetics expert can help you determine whether or not you should get tested, only *you* can make that choice. You should keep in mind that each case is different and highly personal, but here's a synopsis of the National Comprehensive Cancer Network's recommendations. You might consider getting tested:

- If there is a known BRCA1/BRCA2 mutation in the family (or other hereditary breast cancer syndrome).
- If you or a close family member was diagnosed with breast cancer before age forty-five.
- If you or a close family member had two separate breast cancers, with one of the breast cancer diagnoses occurring before age fifty.
- If three or more people in your family (including you) have been diagnosed with breast cancer at any age.
- If two members of your family (including you) were diagnosed with breast cancer before age fifty.
- If you have a family history of breast cancer and an ethnic background associated with a higher mutation frequency, such as people of Ashkenazi Jewish descent.
- If there is ovarian cancer in your family. (This includes fallopian tube and primary peritoneal cancer.)
- If you have a male relative with breast cancer, particularly if there's also more than one person in the family with breast or ovarian cancer.

If you *do* decide to get tested, a blood sample is taken and then sent off to Myriad Genetics, the sole provider of BRACAnalysis, which is the only test for those mutations. Ideally, if someone is going to get tested in your family, it should be the oldest living relative who has had breast or ovarian cancer. For instance, when Lisa first visited her genetics expert, Dr. Morrell, she was told that because of her family history she was a candidate for genetic testing. However, since Lisa's mother, Arlene, had already been diagnosed with breast cancer, Arlene should take the test first. If Arlene tested negative, that would mean the genetic link in

Lisa's maternal side would have ended and Lisa and her brothers could not have that mutation (though Lisa might still have an increased risk of breast cancer because of her family history). If Arlene tested positive, Lisa and her siblings would each have a 50 percent chance of inheriting it from her—and if Lisa did, that would mean she'd have up to an 87 percent chance of developing breast cancer in her lifetime. When Arlene's results came in, she and Lisa returned to Dr. Morrell's office to hear the news: Arlene had tested positive for BRCA2.

Typically, the first person in a family gets a full sequencing, meaning that the test looks at the DNA of both BRCA1 and BRCA2 genes to see if there's a mutation. (There are thousands of possible mutations within these genes, and this test can detect most of them.) For Ashkenazi Jews, the test can focus on three specific mutations that have been passed down for hundreds of years among Jewish individuals. Those mutations are called "founder mutations." Once a genetic mutation has been identified in a family, any relative of that family member can then get tested for that specific site, called single-site testing. Founder mutations and single sites are simpler tests and, therefore, less expensive; a full-sequencing test runs $3,120; a single site is $440; testing for only the three founder mutations common among Ashkenazi Jews is $535. Prices are subject to change, and insurance companies vary their criteria for coverage (see Chapter 7). Results are usually available in less than three weeks.

FINDING OUT THE RESULTS

When testing for BRCA mutations, there are several possible outcomes. Lisa and Mayde, for instance, both tested negative; Rori, Suzanne, and Amy all tested positive. Here's a brief description of each potential result:

Positive: Testing positive means you have a known mutation
for BRCA1 or BRCA2, which in women indicates up to an
87 percent lifetime chance of developing breast cancer and up

to a 44 percent lifetime chance of developing ovarian cancer. That doesn't mean a person with a mutation definitely has 87 percent and 44 percent odds of developing these diseases— one woman might have a 40 percent chance of getting breast cancer, for instance, while another has an 80 percent chance. However, we don't yet have a way to accurately predict a woman's exact odds, so there's no way to tell where on the spectrum she lies. For that reason, experts often play it safe and give the upper ranges of 87 percent and 44 percent. For women, BRCA mutations also slightly increase the risk of melanoma, pancreatic cancer, and other cancers. In men, testing positive puts them at increased risk for prostate and breast cancer, among other cancers. However, it's imperative to note that testing positive does *not* mean that you will definitely get any of these diseases. It also doesn't determine when and where cancer will develop, if it does at all. What it does tell you is that you are at higher risk for cancer, either your mother and/ or your father also had the gene mutation, and your children and siblings have 50-50 odds of being positive, too.

Negative: If a person tests negative for a known mutation in the family, that person has what's called a "true negative," says Alvaro Monteiro, Ph.D., a breast cancer geneticist at the Moffitt Cancer Center in Tampa. "You already know the culprit in your family, and you don't have it," he explains. If all of the risk in your family came from having that gene mutation, your odds of getting breast cancer would be similar to that of the general population. However, it's impossible to know if your family risk is completely caused by the gene or if other environmental and genetic factors are increasing your family's risk, too. "Some research suggests that your risk might still be greater than the average woman's, just not as high as if you had tested positive," adds Dr. Monteiro. "We must wait for long-term prospective studies to completely answer this question."

If a person with a family history of breast or ovarian cancer tests negative and there is no known mutation in the family, those results are even more ambiguous. That person may have a mutation in a part of the BRCA gene not picked up by the test or in a completely different gene altogether. Often, if there's a strong family history, that person will still be treated as a high-risk individual. Also, if indicated by your family history and if you haven't done so already, you might then choose to test for one of the other rare genetic mutations that lead to cancer syndromes such as Cowden syndrome or Li-Fraumeni syndrome (as discussed in Chapter 3).

Variant of uncertain clinical significance: There are normal differences between one person's genes and another's. Sometimes such differences are harmless; other times they are deleterious, which means they can be detrimental to a person's health. A "variant of uncertain clinical significance" result means that there is a difference in a BRCA gene compared with most other people, but the test can't determine whether or not that difference is benign or if it increases a woman's chances of getting breast cancer. Researchers are currently trying to classify every single possible variation in these genes, so women won't get the "We don't know" response, says Dr. Monteiro. But until then, a woman should talk to a genetic counselor to reassess her risk.

It is important to note that sometimes a test can be uninformative. "Uninformative" is a term that means no useful information was derived from the outcome of the test. The first way this result can occur, as discussed above, is when a person tests negative but previous family members also tested negative or they didn't test at all. For instance, say a woman's aunt and mother both died from breast cancer, but they never got tested. Then if that woman tests negative, it's impossible to know whether that means the gene was present in her mother but wasn't passed on, or if something else caused the cancer in her relatives and she may or may not have inherited the risk. The second way a test can be uninformative is when it's a variant of uncertain clinical significance, as described above. What's unfortunate is that such results put a woman back in the same place she started—she still won't be able to estimate her risk.

PSYCHOLOGICAL IMPACT

While the BRCA test itself is simple, finding out the results can be devastating. "The aftermath of testing, regardless of the outcome, can create a lot of psychological distress because women are dealing with the threat of cancer paired with the uncertainty of if and when it'll strike," says Karen Hurley, Ph.D., a psychologist at Memorial Sloan-Kettering Cancer Center in New York City. Emotions can run the gamut. For women who test positive, some are actually relieved, while others believe having the gene mutation is a doomsday sentence. Those who test negative are usually thrilled but sometimes deal with "survivor's guilt" if, say, they're in the clear but their siblings or other family members test positive. Some people who test negative as well as those who get an uninformative result can become incredibly frustrated—they are still living in fear, but are no closer to answering the question of what to do about their risk.

One week after Amy had the mammogram that showed something suspicious, which wound up being nothing, she decided to test for BRCA1, the gene mutation she already knew her mom had. Two weeks later, Amy's genetic counselor called her and said that she had to come back for another visit. Her results were in. "When I got into her office, my counselor said, 'You're positive for BRCA1,'" says Amy. "She then started going over what these results meant and my options, but I couldn't hear what she was saying. I felt like I was watching a *Charlie Brown* cartoon where the teacher speaks, but the kids hear only that garbled, incoherent voice. All I could think was that I wanted to get out of the appointment and not deal with this. For so long, I had thought I had a high risk for breast cancer. Now I knew without a doubt that my fears were confirmed. It was too much to handle."

Mayde, on the other hand, tested negative. But she, too, was completely floored by her results. "From the day my mother's breast surgeon shook his finger at me and told me I had to always be careful because my mother had battled breast cancer, I was worried I'd follow in my mother's footsteps. Sure enough, when I was forty-four, one of my mammograms came back showing microcalcifications in both breasts, which signified I needed further testing. I went in for a breast MRI at my husband's radiology practice and had a biopsy of one area that revealed I had atypical lobular hyperplasia (ALH). Three months later, I found out that the cells had proliferated and progressed to lobular carcinoma in situ (LCIS) as well as atypical ductal hyperplasia (ADH), both of which raised my risk of getting breast cancer significantly. A few of my doctors told me I had "pre-cancer." After that diagnosis, I ran home and grabbed my mother's original pathology report that I had always kept in my underwear drawer, just in case. My report mirrored my mother's word for word. She also had "widespread LCIS" and "ADH" primarily in her left breast, just like I had. And so when my mother and I both tested negative, I was relieved but stunned and even more confused. I thought, 'How could there not be a genetic link?'"

A SINGLE GIRL'S PERSPECTIVE

While genetic testing can have a huge impact on anyone, choosing to have genetic testing means something very different for, say, a single woman versus someone who is married with kids. "Potentially having a genetic mutation is unnerving enough, but it can be a lot worse when the rest of your life isn't settled," says Lindsay Avner, who, after finding out at twenty-two that she was positive for BRCA1, founded Bright Pink, a nonprofit organization geared toward young women who are at high risk for breast and/or ovarian cancer. "We'd all like to fall in love naturally and have kids on our own time line, but many high-risk women might feel an enormous pressure to hurry up and meet Mr. Right, get married, and have children. For us, the gene not only threatens our risk for getting cancer, but it also has the potential to threaten who we wind up with and whether or not we have kids. Someone who already has a family doesn't have to deal with those issues."

THE RIPPLE EFFECT

Genetic testing, especially if the results are positive, can open up a can of worms within a family. When a person finds out she has a genetic mutation, emotions can run high not only for her but also for her relatives who might be affected. It can help to talk to an expert about the best way to broach the topic.

After Suzanne initially spoke with Mayde at her dance studio, she eventually saw a genetic counselor, went through with testing, and found out she was positive for BRCA2. Almost immediately, she felt a responsibility to share her results with her family because she knew they could be affected, too. "When I told my sister, she snapped 'What's this now?'" recalls Suzanne. "She seemed annoyed with me—it was just another thing *she'd* have to deal with because *I* decided to get tested. My brother's response was, 'Oh well, that's too bad. But I don't have breasts or ovaries. I'm not getting tested.' I could see I was getting nowhere, so I suggested they both go on the FORCE website and read about BRCA themselves. Once they learned about it and realized the repercussions of having the gene mutation, they both changed their tunes. My sister got tested first and, thankfully, was negative. My brother realized that he could have the mutation as easily as a woman could and that he could have passed it along to his two daughters. He tested next and was positive (as, we later found out, was one of his daughters). Now my family is so grateful that I initiated all of this. Well, most of my family is. After my eighty-year-old aunt, the only survivor of my mother's immediate family, tested positive, only her daughter decided to get tested. The rest of my cousins, all stubborn Italian men, have yet to do so. It scares me because they all have daughters who could be at risk. I try to talk to my cousins and have written them e-mails and letters, but I haven't heard back from them. There's nothing more I can do."

interpreting your risk

Finding out your risk is one thing, but how you perceive it, in some ways, is even more important when it comes down to deciding what to do next. One woman with a BRCA1 mutation might view a possible 87 percent chance of getting breast cancer as a death sentence. Another might look at the 13-percent-or-greater odds of not getting breast cancer and hope for the best. It's a question of how risk adverse you are.

Amy and Rori tested positive for BRCA1; Suzanne tested positive for BRCA2. Though their results had similar potential impact on their risk, they each dealt with the news differently. When her genetic counselor told her the results, Rori says she literally broke down and started crying. "To me, having the gene meant I was almost certain to get cancer during my lifetime," she says. "I'm usually optimistic, but at this point I felt sick to my stomach, shocked, and a complete sense of sadness. And for the rest of the week, I was so devastated that I couldn't even leave my house." Suzanne, on the other hand, was actually relieved that she tested positive. "I knew I was at risk, and testing positive just validated my suspicions," Suzanne says. "I now had the proof I needed to move forward and do something about it."

Amy says she was completely overwhelmed after learning her results. And since she was so reluctant to even talk about her cancer risk in the first place, she barely dealt with the implications of her genetic mutation. "When I first found out I was positive, I wasn't ready to act on it, so I tucked my results away in a drawer and didn't look at them for nine months," she says. "I also didn't follow my genetic counselor's instructions to increase surveillance and actually missed my mammogram that year. Instead, I spent hours lurking on the computer, finding out everything I could about BRCA and my options. I know that skipping screening might not have been smart, but the only thing that gave me any peace was gathering my facts so that I could figure out what my next move would be."

As for Lisa and Mayde, they both tested negative for BRCA1 and BRCA2. However, neither thought that meant they were out of the woods. "I still had a family history and previous biopsies that one expert said put my risk at about 30 percent," says Lisa, who took the test after her mother, Arlene, found out she was positive for BRCA2. "To me, those are odds I didn't want to take. And though I was lucky I didn't have the mutation my mother had, I couldn't help but think, 'Who knows what other hereditary or environmental factors could be at play? What if there's another gene that just hasn't been discovered yet?'"

Mayde adds: "Of course, I was happy that my negative test meant I wouldn't pass a mutated gene on to my kids and that my risk for ovarian cancer wasn't elevated, but it didn't change my perceived risk of breast cancer. I still had so many other risk factors that were adding up. My breast cells had already proliferated considerably, and I started seeing my medical history as a flow chart, a continuum. My next stop was breast cancer."

Dealing with these issues can be daunting, which is why you should never hesitate to call your genetic counselor or doctor with questions. Also, in some cases a woman might seek professional help from a psychologist, particularly if she finds that her focus on her risk becomes all-consuming. However, sometimes the best emotional support comes from women who have already been through it all. "When I found out how high my risk was, I really wanted to talk to someone in the same situation as I was," says Mayde, who didn't meet the other four women in this book until after she had already had a prophylactic mastectomy. "There were plenty of organizations for survivors of breast cancer, but I just couldn't relate to those women because I didn't have the disease. Then, by randomly searching on Google, I discovered FORCE, a nonprofit organization that caters to women who have an increased risk for breast and ovarian cancer. I searched the message boards and found so many women who were just like me—other previvors who had a predisposition for developing breast cancer but didn't have the illness. It was so reassuring to know I wasn't alone." Suzanne, as the last of the five women to face her risk, feels especially blessed that she found an incredible support network near her own home. "The most help I got emotionally was from pouring my heart out to Lisa, Mayde, Amy, and Rori. As supportive as my husband and other friends were, they couldn't really understand what I was going through in the same way these women could. My psychological counseling came from those four girls."

While finding out one's risk can be frightening, many women ultimately find it empowering. After letting the news of her results sink in for a few days, Rori began to view them differently. "I started thinking 'Knowledge is power' and became enamored with this enlightening information I had been given. I told myself, 'I'm not sick. I'm healthy. I might have a very high risk for getting cancer, but at least now I can choose to do something about it.'" And Lisa, Mayde, Amy, Rori, and Suzanne each decided that they would.

weighing the options

NONSURGICAL

Once you've determined that you've got a good chance of getting breast cancer in your lifetime (and, for women with a BRCA gene mutation, ovarian cancer), you have two choices: Either you do nothing and hope you beat the odds, or you take action and try to defy your fate. Making these decisions can be distressing and complicated, which is why women often rely on a team of experts such as surgeons, oncologists, gynecologists, genetics experts, and psychologists to help them figure out what to do.

Mayde, who is always thorough when making *any* decision, says that weighing her options consumed her life for months. "I was a madwoman, reading everything and anything I could find online, printing out dozens of articles," she says. "I'd stay up doing research until three a.m. Then I'd go to bed, wake up at six a.m., and I'd be right back on the computer the second the kids left for school." During this time, Mayde also saw a psychologist, a genetic counselor, an oncologist, and multiple breast surgeons and plastic surgeons. "I was on a mission—I had to be armed with every ounce of information I might need so I could make an informed decision," she says. "I needed a team of experts to help me through this maze."

This chapter explores the nonsurgical options available to women who have an elevated risk of getting breast cancer; the next chapter looks at surgical alternatives. Each choice has its pros and cons with different issues to consider. This breakdown is intended to give you a head start in figuring out which path is best for you. And for a glimpse at what might be available in the future, see Chapter 14.

lifestyle changes

Many women who have elevated odds of getting breast cancer make lifestyle changes that might lower their risk. These may include cutting back on alcohol, maintaining a healthy weight, and exercising more frequently. While such changes won't have as large an effect on risk as some other options will, experts say they can only help. For instance, after her mother was diagnosed with breast cancer, Lisa started working out religiously and paying attention to any new reports that came out regarding the disease. "When the experts said to eat blueberries, I ate blueberries," she says. "When they said to try soy products, I did. And then when they said to stop eating soy because it stimulates estrogen production, I stopped. I drove myself crazy trying to follow all of the varying advice out there, especially considering how often the news changes." Rori says that when she found out she had a high risk for cancer, she started taking more vitamins, meditating, exercising more frequently, and trying basically anything that might make her lifestyle even healthier than it already was. Mayde even went so far as to enroll in high-risk surveillance programs, through which experts gave her nutritional advice, put her on a vitamin regimen, and closely monitored her cysts.

But while these women also eventually opted for a more dramatic means of lowering their odds, some women decide not to do anything to counter their risk. Rori's sister Nancie, for instance, doesn't want to face her risk even though there's a known mutation in her family and her mother and other sister, Lynne, both battled ovarian cancer. "Nancie knows she's at high risk, but she's not going to do anything about it," says Rori. "She doesn't go to doctors, and she doesn't get mammograms or even do breast self-exams. She is not having genetic testing or counseling. Nancie probably doesn't think she'll get cancer, and she figures that if she does she'll just deal with it. She lives her life. Period. End of story. But that's her personal decision and I have to respect that—she has her way of reacting to her risk and I have mine."

increased surveillance

The whole idea behind surveillance is using various tests and screening methods to catch cancer in its earliest, most treatable stage. While surveillance can't prevent cancer, it *can* detect it early and possibly spare a woman from having to go through chemotherapy or worse. In fact, according to the American Cancer Society, the five-year survival rate for women who detect breast cancer before it has spread is 98 percent. "Often the earlier you catch cancer, the better the odds for survival," explains Kathryn Evers, M.D., director of breast imaging at Fox Chase Cancer Center in Philadelphia. And that's especially the case among younger women who tend to get tumors that are more aggressive.

Though national breast cancer screening guidelines vary by organization, here's what the American Cancer Society recommends for women with average risk:

- Yearly mammograms starting at age forty.
- Clinical breast exam (CBE) every three years for women in their twenties and thirties and every year for women forty and older.

- Breast self-exam (BSE) is an option for women beginning in their twenties. Women should know how their breasts feel normally and immediately report any breast change to their health care providers.
- MRI is not recommended for women in this category.

High-risk women might want to start such screening much earlier, and in the case of clinical breast exams, more often. Also, the American Cancer Society recommends that they add yearly MRI to their regimen. Work with your doctor to develop a screening regimen appropriate for you.

Here's a breakdown of what each of these surveillance methods entail:

Breast Self-Exams

No studies have shown that breast self-exams can lower the risk of dying from breast cancer. And for that reason, some national organizations now recommend that women no longer do them. However, says Dr. Evers, the truth is many women discover their own lumps. "While there isn't any great data about breast self-exams, if you happen to detect cancer by doing one, that's a *good* thing," she says. "Breast self-exams are free and easy, and if you do find something, your doctor will help determine whether or not you need further testing or a biopsy."

Mayde saw firsthand the role breast self-exams can play in fighting cancer. Her mother, Blossom, performed them religiously and often found cysts that her breast surgeon then aspirated. All were benign until the last cyst she found—it turned out she had breast cancer. "I believe that my mother's vigilance really paid off because she caught a cancer that had been missed by her mammogram," says Mayde. "If she hadn't done her breast exams, who knows what might have happened? She possibly saved her own life."

The American Cancer Society says that doing breast self-exams is a personal choice, one they don't encourage or dissuade a woman from making. If you do choose to do breast self-exams, they should never take the place of routine clinical breast exams or mammograms. Also, always try to do them at the same time every month when your breasts aren't tender (i.e., not directly before or during your period). Many women prefer to perform the exam in the shower—it's convenient and the soapy water makes it easier for their fingers to glide over their breasts. Ask your doctor or nurse practitioner to teach you the correct technique (for a quick tutorial, you can also check out www.komen.org/bse). Basically, you should look for any changes in the size and shape of your breasts, lumps, painful areas, changes in skin color or texture, crusting or bleeding nipples, discharge, or anything out of the ordinary.

Clinical Breast Exams

While a woman knows her own breasts and can detect changes by doing self-exams, sometimes a doctor can better determine when something is outside the range of normal. A doctor will typically first look for abnormalities in the breasts' size, shape, or color. Then, using the tips of her fingers, she will palpate (touch) the breasts and under the arms, looking for any suspicious lumps or thickening of the skin. Sometimes such exams can find cancers that aren't detected by a mammogram.

Mammograms

Mammograms are X-rays of the breasts that identify changes (including tumors) in breast tissue. They have traditionally been the gold standard of breast cancer detection and have been proven to reduce the mortality rate of the disease. Mammograms detect subtle changes in the breast that can't be felt, as well as microcalcifications (small clusters of calcium) that indicate heightened cell activity and that might signify that breast cancer is present. Like any screening tool, mammograms aren't perfect—they can miss up to 20 percent of breast cancers, according to the National Cancer Institute. They can also lead to false positives, which means the mammogram identifies a suspicious change that looks like cancer but isn't. This, in turn, may lead to unnecessary biopsies, anxiety, loss of time at work or with family, and additional costs.

There are two kinds of mammograms: traditional (analog) and digital. Neither affects how the mammogram is performed from the patient's point of view; they just differ in how the images are acquired and stored. With traditional mammograms, the images are captured and stored on a piece of film, while with digital they are captured and stored electronically on a computer. The main benefit of digital is that radiologists can adjust the image of the breast tissue (just like you can remove red eye in a digital picture or enlarge it). This can allow for better detection of slight differences that might indicate microcalcifications or early masses.

In terms of effectiveness, a major national trial found that while digital mammograms have no benefit over traditional mammograms for the average woman, they *do* detect more cancers in women who fall into any of the following categories:

- Women under age fifty
- Those of any age with very dense breasts
- Premenopausal or perimenopausal women of any age

For Mayde, traditional mammograms never picked up any microcalcifications, but her very first digital mammogram did. That finding eventually led to her diagnosis of atypical ductal hyperplasia, which her doctors told her was pre-cancer. However, keep in mind that *any* mammogram—digital or traditional—is better than none. If digital mammograms aren't offered in your area, it's still important to keep up with regular screenings. There might be plenty of excuses not to—mammograms can be uncomfortable or even painful for some women (which is why experts recommend not getting mammograms right before or during your period, when your breasts might be more tender). Also, some women might fear the results so much that they bypass the test altogether. Yet the benefits of mammograms are too great to ignore. "Yes, they flatten your breast like a pancake and waiting for the results can be absolutely terrifying, but I always figured all of that was worth it if the mammogram possibly found early-stage breast cancer," says Lisa. "I understand wanting to avoid mammograms, but I felt like if I did have breast cancer, I'd rather catch it early and fight it than face the alternative. I saw what chemo did to my mother. I saw her eventually die a horrible death. I would do anything to avoid that."

In 2009, the U.S. Preventive Services Task Force sparked an immediate debate when they started recommending that women begin getting mammograms at age fifty every two years instead of at age forty every year or two. As this recommendation does not apply to very high risk women, their reasoning was that women in their forties are not in great danger of developing breast cancer. Also, they explained, mammograms among this age group can lead to many false positives and unnecessary biopsies. The release of these new guidelines greatly angered many doctors, researchers, and breast cancer organizations (let alone a countless number of women who have been affected by the disease). They argue that mammograms have detected cancer in many women in their forties and that this demographic still deserves the right to be screened. Also, they fear that these new guidelines might lead to insurance companies denying coverage of mammograms among women in this age bracket. For such reasons, many organizations such as the American Cancer Society still recommend mammograms every year starting at age forty.

MRI (Magnetic Resonance Imaging)
MRIs are the newest step in screening for high-risk women. An MRI uses a magnetic field and radio waves to produce many images of a

woman's breasts. During the procedure, the patient lies facedown on the scanning table. The breasts hang into a hollow in the table, which has coils that detect the radiofrequency signal. The entire table then enters a tubelike machine that contains the magnet. After the radiologist takes an initial series of images, the patient may be injected with a contrast agent that can help detect any tumors. Extra images are then taken. The entire imaging session lasts up to one hour, and aside from the injection, the whole process is painless. However, it can be uncomfortable for people who are claustrophobic.

The biggest plus to getting an MRI is that it's an extremely sensitive test that finds most invasive cancers. It can also detect how far the breast cancer has spread better than mammograms can. However, MRIs don't pick up microcalcifications and, because they're so sensitive, they often lead to false positives that can result in unnecessary biopsies (especially at centers that have less experience with the technique).

Experts recommend that women with a high risk for breast cancer get yearly MRIs as well as mammograms. When actress Christina Applegate was diagnosed with breast cancer in 2008, she publicly credited MRI for catching the cancer early and possibly saving her life.

Ultrasound

Ultrasound, also called sonography, is an imaging technique in which high-frequency sound waves are bounced off tissues and internal organs. Their echoes produce a picture called a sonogram. "From the patient's perspective, the process is the same as when you're pregnant," explains Amy. "Though looking at a baby is a lot more fun." Ultrasounds, usually used to evaluate a mass found on either a mammogram or during a breast exam, help distinguish between solid tumors and fluid-filled cysts. One study by the American College of Radiology Imaging Network (ACRIN) found that screening ultrasounds combined with mammograms pick up 28 percent more cancers in women with an increased risk for breast cancer than mammography alone. However, like MRIs, ultrasounds may not pick up microcalcifications. Also, as ultrasounds are extremely dependent on the skill of the technician performing them, again, this can result in a lot of false negatives, false positives, and unnecessary biopsies.

CAD (Computer Aided Detection)

Many breast-imaging centers now have computer programs which, when used with mammograms, can detect up to 20 percent more cancers than mammograms alone. After the radiologist has reviewed the imaging results, he lets the CAD evaluate them. The CAD software highlights any areas of the breast that might look suspicious, and the radiologist then determines if any of those areas need further examination. It's like getting a second opinion, but from a computer instead of from another person. The CAD program may be particularly useful in detecting subtle changes and microcalcifications, though it's important to weigh any benefits against possible drawbacks. While some studies have found CAD a useful tool, others have found that it increases the false-positive rate without finding a significant number of cancers.

You might also hear about CAD being used with MRI, but this is different from CAD used with mammograms. These computer systems help radiologists determine the size and location of cancers found with MRI.

Ovarian Cancer Screening

For women who test positive for BRCA1 or BRCA2, breast cancer is not the only disease they have to contend with. "When I found out my risk for breast cancer, I also learned that I had up to a 44 percent chance of getting ovarian cancer during my lifetime compared to the average woman's risk of 1.4 percent," says Rori, who has a BRCA1 mutation. "That statistic is what scared me the most. With breast cancer, at least you can sometimes find a lump. But ovarian cancer is commonly called the 'silent killer'—women like my mother often don't detect any symptoms until it's too late." In fact, according to the Ovarian Cancer National Alliance, about 55 percent of people who get the disease die from it within five years. The reason: Ovarian cancer is usually diagnosed at an advanced stage, past the point it can be effectively treated. If ovarian cancer is found early and treated before it has spread, the five-year survival rate is higher than 90 percent. However, less than 20 percent of all ovarian cancers are found at this early stage.

In some ways, the term "silent killer" is a misnomer, because there actually *are* signs of ovarian cancer. One way to possibly catch the disease earlier is seeing your doctor if you've had any of the following symptoms for more than a few weeks (symptoms that are not normal for *you*): bloating, pelvic or abdominal pain, difficulty eating or feeling full quickly, and urinary symptoms (urgency and frequency). However, many patients don't mention these symptoms to their doctors because they write them off to other medical conditions such as their menstrual cycles or gas pains. And even when patients do mention the symptoms to their doctors, many physicians don't consider ovarian cancer in the realm of possibilities because the disease is much less common than breast cancer (one woman in seventy-one gets the disease during her lifetime versus one in eight for breast cancer).

Other screening methods for ovarian cancer exist, though none has been proven to greatly affect the odds of catching the disease early. For high-risk women, experts recommend screening every six months starting at age thirty, or five to ten years earlier than the earliest age anyone in your family was diagnosed with ovarian cancer. The options include:

- **Pelvic exam:** A doctor will feel the ovaries and other nearby organs for irregularities, such as enlargement.
- **Transvaginal ultrasound:** A doctor inserts a small probe into the vagina that transmits sound waves. These waves create a

snapshot of the ovaries, which the doctor can then view on a computer screen to look for signs of ovarian cancer. However, most abnormalities that are detected are not cancer. In turn, this test can lead to a lot of false positives.

- **Blood test for CA-125:** CA-125, a protein in our bodies, is sometimes elevated when ovarian cancer is present. The drawback is that a lot of other much more common medical conditions such as fibroids, endometriosis, and pregnancy can also increase CA-125 levels.

chemoprevention

The National Cancer Institute (NCI) defines chemoprevention as "the use of drugs, vitamins, or other agents to try to reduce the risk of, or delay the development or recurrence of, cancer." Currently, there are a few options available to women looking to reduce their risk of breast cancer, though none is perfect. "It's a balancing act," says Leslie Ford, M.D., associate director of clinical research at the NCI's Division of Cancer Prevention. "We've found some drugs that help decrease a woman's odds of getting breast cancer, but each comes with its own risks. You have to discuss with your doctor whether or not chemoprevention is right for you." Also, keep in mind that chemoprevention reduces risk, but it doesn't eliminate it. If you choose this option, surveillance is still important.

Here's what's available:

SERMs

We all have cell proteins in our bodies called estrogen receptors. Estrogen binds to those receptors and, in turn, may cause the cells to grow and multiply. However, there's a class of drugs called selective estrogen receptor modulators (SERMs) that bind to these receptors instead, and seem to block estrogen from attaching in breast tissue. SERMs don't decrease the amount of estrogen in a person's breasts—experts believe they just limit the effect the hormone has. SERMs also have different effects on different organs. In breast tissue, SERMs appear to stop the effects of estrogen, while in the uterus, bone, and blood vessels, they can actually mimic the effects of the hormone, causing some beneficial side effects as well as some unwanted ones. Currently, there are two SERMs approved by the Food and Drug Administration (FDA)—tamoxifen and raloxifene—for women who have an increased risk for developing breast cancer.

TAMOXIFEN

Tamoxifen is a drug that blocks some of the effects estrogen has on breast tissue. It was originally used to prevent a recurrence in someone who has already had breast cancer. However, when results from a national study showed that women are 49 percent less likely to develop breast cancer if they take tamoxifen, the FDA approved the drug for breast cancer prevention in women thirty-five or older in 1998. Women on tamoxifen, which is available as a generic, take one pill daily for five years. However, if your risk comes from having a BRCA1 mutation, tamoxifen might not be for you. Women like Rori and Amy who are BRCA1 positive are more likely to get estrogen-receptor-negative breast cancer (which means the cancer cells do not need estrogen to grow), and tamoxifen only seems to decrease risk in estrogen-receptor-*positive* tumors. There is some evidence that tamoxifen might benefit women who have a BRCA2 mutation, but more research needs to be done.

Because tamoxifen has side effects such as an increased risk of endometrial cancer and blood clotting (mainly in postmenopausal women),

women should consider the possible benefits and risks of tamoxifen when deciding whether or not it is right for them. For instance, women who already have a risk for blood clots—such as diabetics and smokers—might not be good candidates. Other side effects include vaginal dryness, vaginal discharge, leg cramps, hot flashes, and bladder problems. Many women believe that tamoxifen can cause weight gain and depression, though no studies have ever shown that to be the case. According to Dr. Ford, any accounts of these effects are anecdotal, but it's impossible to know if those women gained weight and became depressed because of the drug or if they would have experienced those symptoms anyway.

None of the women in this book opted to take tamoxifen, each for different reasons. Rori and Amy both have a BRCA1 mutation, which, as just explained, possibly means they wouldn't reap any benefits from the drug. Mayde already has an elevated risk for leg cramps and blood clots, so tamoxifen was contraindicated in her case, while Lisa's doctor told her that she wasn't a candidate and strongly suggested surveillance instead. Suzanne says a 49 percent risk reduction simply wasn't satisfactory to her—she, as well as the other women, wanted an option that would eliminate as much risk as possible.

RALOXIFENE

Like tamoxifen, raloxifene (brand name: Evista) also blocks the effect of estrogen on breast tissue. In 2007, the FDA approved it for breast cancer risk reduction in postmenopausal women with an increased risk for breast cancer (it had already been approved for osteoporosis prevention and treatment among this same age group). A large NCI-sponsored study comparing the effectiveness of this drug and tamoxifen found that, in a long-term follow-up, raloxifene was about 76 percent as effective as tamoxifen in reducing invasive breast cancer risk. In other words, while tamoxifen lowers risk about 49 percent, raloxifene lowers it about 37 percent. Since the study did not include premenopausal women or specifically look at women with BRCA mutations, it is unknown whether the drug will have similar effects on these particular demographics. (All of the women in this book were premenopausal, so they couldn't have taken raloxifene even if they had wanted to do so.) Like tamoxifen, raloxifene is a pill taken daily for five years.

In terms of side effects, the NCI trial found that compared with tamoxifen, raloxifene has considerably lower risks of certain side effects such as uterine and endometrial cancer and blood clots (although the risk of blood clots was still higher than normal). Women did cite symptoms such as hot flashes, vaginal dryness, vaginal discharge, pain during intercourse, weight gain, and bone and muscle problems.

CHEMOPREVENTION FOR OVARIAN CANCER

Studies have shown that taking birth control pills for five or more years over a lifetime may decrease a woman's odds of getting ovarian cancer by 50 percent or higher. However, this statistic refers to the general population; other studies conflict over whether or not this benefit applies to women with BRCA mutations. Oral contraceptives *may* increase the odds of getting breast cancer, so talk to your doctor about whether or not you should consider taking them. After Suzanne had her prophylactic mastectomy, she asked her breast surgeon about oral contraceptives. "I had already nearly eliminated my risk for breast cancer, but I wasn't ready to have my ovaries removed to reduce my risk for ovarian cancer," says Suzanne. "My doctor said that taking the Pill was 'better than nothing' and so I figured, 'Why not?' Until I'm ready for the surgery, at least I feel like I'm doing something to protect myself."

the next step

While plenty of previvors stick with the options described in this chapter, some get to the point where they want to do whatever will reduce their breast cancer risk (and for those with a BRCA mutation, ovarian cancer risk) the most. That brings us to prophylactic surgeries, which are explained in the next chapter.

CHAPTER SIX

weighing the options

SURGICAL

Many women with an elevated breast cancer risk would never consider prophylactic surgeries as a means to beat their odds. Some, like Lisa, Mayde, Amy, and Rori, choose surveillance for years, even decades, before turning to this measure as a last resort. And then there are those who, once they start dealing with their risk, almost immediately know they want to have surgery. Suzanne, for instance, knew what action she'd take before she even went through with genetic testing. "For me, I couldn't get tested and then figure out 'Now what?' depending on the results," she says. "I kind of did things backward—I knew that if I tested negative, I would stick with vigilant surveillance and do nothing else. But I also had to have a game plan for what I'd do if I tested positive. That plan was to hit my risk as hard as I could, and I had already learned that having a prophylactic mastectomy was my best shot at preventing breast cancer. By the time I was figuring out my options, Mayde had already had her surgery. One day in my dance studio, she gave me a 'show-and-tell,' and I thought, 'Wow, if her kind of reconstruction is an option, I'll sign up for that.' So I decided then and there that if I tested positive, I'd have the same exact surgery that Mayde had. I never looked back."

Here's a look at what prophylactic surgeries are available to women today.

prophylactic mastectomy

Studies have shown that a bilateral prophylactic mastectomy—the removal of both breasts in a woman who doesn't have breast cancer—can reduce a woman's risk of getting breast cancer by at least 90 percent. It doesn't completely eliminate risk because surgeons can't be sure they remove all breast tissue. (Tissue can reach the armpit, as high as the collarbone, and as low as the abdomen.)

Of course, prophylactic mastectomies are not for everyone. The Society of Surgical Oncology states that this surgery is only appropriate for people who have a known BRCA mutation or a mutation of a breast cancer susceptibly gene; a strong family history of breast and/or ovarian cancer; or atypical hyperplasia or lobular carcinoma in situ (especially when paired with a strong family history of breast cancer). But even if your risk indicates that you should consider the surgery, choosing to actually go through with it is an extremely difficult decision, one that women often reach after months, if not years, of contemplating whether or not it's right for them.

When Rori first found out she had tested positive for BRCA1, she met with her genetic counselor and a gynecologic oncologist to talk about her options. The oncologist told her that along with having her ovaries removed she should contemplate a prophylactic mastectomy. "I almost fell off my chair when he said that," recalls Rori. "I was like, 'Hello, are you kidding me? I'm a mother. I'm a wife. I'm healthy.' Having a mastectomy wasn't even a blip on my radar. It seemed so drastic to me. There was no way I was going to have what I then saw as a mutilating surgery. I was set on doing surveillance."

For a long time, Lisa felt the same way. Once she found out she did not have the BRCA mutation her mother had, she would get a mammogram and ultrasound once a year, but that's it. "I kind of kicked back because I felt like I was doing enough surveillance to protect myself," Lisa says. But then her mother passed away and, eight months later, Lisa had a mammogram that picked up two masses in her right breast—the first time a mammogram found something that Lisa hadn't discovered herself. Her oncologist suggested they watch the masses. Six months later, they had changed slightly. "At that point, my oncologist suggested I keep watching these lumps, but I was just sickened by the whole thing," says Lisa. "I said to myself, 'How many times are we going to go through this? I'm done watching. I've been watching my whole life.' That's when I went to a breast surgeon, the same surgeon who performed my previous biopsies and my mother's lumpectomy, and I asked him, 'What are my options if I want to get rid of my risk as much as possible?' (I just couldn't bring myself to say the word 'mastectomy.') He said, 'You could get a prophylactic mastectomy, but that's a very personal decision. There's no guideline out there that says you should get this, but many women are doing it because they just don't want to live with their risk anymore.' I thought he was going to say that I was crazy for even thinking about having the surgery, but he was very understanding. He had seen what I had gone through with my mother and my previous biopsies. He understood why I was so frightened. I immediately started doing research to see if there was a procedure I would consider."

TYPES OF MASTECTOMIES

Years ago, a mastectomy meant the removal of the entire breast along with lymph nodes and chest muscles. Mayde recalls that her mother's mastectomy in the 1970s left her "flat as a board with a railroad-type stitch over her chest." Fortunately, women today have many more options than their mothers did, and these radical mastectomies are rarely performed anymore. Instead, surgeons focus not only on preventing cancer but also on improving the aesthetic outcome. "Surgical techniques have advanced to the point that a woman can consider a prophylactic mastectomy with reconstruction knowing that, in the end, she will still look whole and have natural-looking breasts," says Frank DellaCroce, M.D., co-director of the Center for Restorative Breast Surgery in New Orleans.

Today, women who opt for prophylactic mastectomies typically have a **total mastectomy (also called a simple mastectomy),** which means the entire breast, including the nipple and areola, is removed. Women who have this kind of surgery can have reconstruction immediately, down the road, or never. (For women who opt for the latter two options, the doctors stitch them up. Then, if and when the patient decides to have reconstruction, the surgeons can use tissue flaps or expanders to stretch the skin. These techniques are described later in this chapter.)

For women who are having immediate reconstruction, doctors will perform a **skin-sparing mastectomy,** which means the skin is preserved and only the nipple and areola are removed. Basically, the breast surgeon scoops out the breast tissue, so to speak, and creates a pocket that the plastic surgeon can then fill with an implant or tissue from another part of the body (see the section on reconstruction later in this chapter). Studies have shown that preserving the skin does not increase the risk of breast cancer. However, it can greatly improve the final appearance of a woman's breasts after surgery.

NIPPLE SPARING

For many women who have decided to have a prophylactic mastectomy, one of their biggest decisions is whether or not to preserve the nipple. Nipple-sparing procedures are becoming more common. Yet they remain controversial. On the one hand, nipples contain some breast cells, so theoretically keeping them could translate to a minimally higher risk. Some doctors figure if you're going to have the preventative surgery, you might as well remove as much tissue as possible. Other experts say that women should at least know that nipple sparing is available as it appears to be a safe technique (even for some patients who have already been diagnosed with breast cancer). "Women should have a range of options when considering a prophylactic mastectomy, and nipple sparing is a reasonable one," says Steven Narod, M.D., one of the leading BRCA researchers in the world and director of the Familial Breast Cancer Research Unit at Women's College Research Institute in Toronto. "In any case, the risk of breast cancer for a woman with a BRCA mutation who had a nipple-sparing mastectomy is much less than that of an average woman with no mutation."

Another factor to consider is that preserving the nipple does improve cosmetic outcome, which, for some, is more important than a hypothetical risk. In fact, some women—like the ones in this book—say that if nipple sparing weren't an option, they wouldn't have gone through with a prophylactic mastectomy at all. "I figured that since I was healthy and didn't actually have breast cancer, having a surgery that decreased my risk way below that of the average woman was enough," explains Amy. "It was important to me that when I looked in the mirror, my breasts still looked like they were mine. I imagined that it would be a lot harder for me psychologically if they didn't."

If you decide to keep your nipples, the surgeon will remove breast tissue through an incision under the breast or on it. The nipple, areola, and skin remain intact. During the surgery, the doctor usually removes tissue and milk ducts in the nipple and has it immediately evaluated by a pathologist. If the report shows the cells are cancerous, then the nipple and areola will be removed. In very rare cases, typically when a large-breasted woman opts to reduce her cup size, the doctor will perform a nipple transplant—the nipple is completely removed from the breast and then regrafted back onto the breast. Though, at that point, many doctors prefer to just re-create the nipple from scratch (see section below on nipple reconstruction).

RISKS OF SURGERY

Prophylactic mastectomies are considered very safe, but, as with any surgery, there are risks involved. These include bleeding, swelling and pain, excessive scar tissue, infection, changes in nipple and breast sensation, fatigue, the need for additional surgeries, and various problems with anesthesia. For instance, a week after her surgery, Lisa had to have another operation to stop some internal bleeding near the surgical site. Though Lisa never found out exactly what caused the bleeding, her doctors think that maybe the removal of her surgical drain created a tear. "Everything turned out to be fine and I was still happy I had the operation, but it certainly wasn't a piece of cake," Lisa says. Amy also had to have a second surgery when her surgical stitches opened up. However, it's important to note that many patients will recover with little or no complications.

After a mastectomy, patients often experience loss of sensation in their breasts, and they will no longer be able to breast-feed. The surgery is irreversible, but it doesn't completely eliminate breast cancer risk. It reduces the odds by at least 90 percent, but it's impossible for surgeons to know if they have removed every cell of breast tissue.

reconstruction options

Regardless of the type of mastectomy you choose, you'll have many options if you want to have reconstruction. Not all women take this next step. Some forgo reconstruction and might use prostheses (shaped mounds made of silicone, foam, or other material) to simply fill their bras. However, if you do decide to go ahead with reconstruction, which most women do, the first choice is whether to have implants, a flap surgery (which uses your own tissue to re-create the breasts), or a combination of the two. Here's an overview of each option:

IMPLANTS

Saline Versus Silicone

Nowadays, many surgeons prefer silicone implants over saline because the gel-filled material looks more natural and has less rippling and distortion than the water balloon–like effect of saline. However, others are still wary of silicone—in 1992, the Food and Drug Administration (FDA) removed silicone gel–filled breast implants from the market because of the lack of data to support their safety and effectiveness. (Silicone was still permitted for breast reconstruction after mastectomies.) Yet no studies showed such harm, and in 2006 the FDA approved silicone breast implants manufactured by the companies Mentor and Allergan. People still might choose saline (which, ironically, comes in a silicone shell) because they're anxious about silicone and they don't trust the science, but most experts agree that silicone has a better cosmetic outcome.

Expanders Versus One-Stage Surgeries

Once you decide what type of implant you want, your next decision is which surgical procedure to choose. With expanders, a silicone-shelled balloon temporarily goes under the skin and muscle right after the mastectomy (or whenever the patient decides to have reconstruction). Over several months, a doctor or nurse will inject the expander with saline through a valve in the device, thereby stretching the skin and chest wall to create a pocket for the implant. Then, in an outpatient surgery, the expanders are replaced with the permanent saline or silicone implant.

Expanders are the cornerstone of implant surgeries, and they allow surgeons to fine-tune the results of the reconstruction. However, they entail a lengthy and uncomfortable process, says Dr. DellaCroce. "You have to get stuck with a needle every time the expanders are filled up, and the fluid can create a lot of pressure on your rib cage and chest wall, kind of like getting braces on your teeth tightened," he says.

Newer direct-to-implant techniques remove the need for traditional expanders. One option you might want to ask your doctor about is permanent expanders, which are basically adjustable implants that remain in place once they're fully expanded. Even more commonly, some surgeons now use acellular skin grafts to extend the muscle and create a pocket for the implant (which essentially accomplishes what expanders do, though in one step). These materials include AlloDerm, derived from human tissue, and Strattice, derived from pigskin. They give the implant more padding and help hold it in place like, as one expert puts it, "a scaffold." They also give the breasts a more natural look because the extra layer between the implant and the skin makes any irregularities in the implant less noticeable. Usually, with this nipple-sparing procedure, there is no visible scarring since the incision is typically underneath the breast fold.

Many women who prefer the one-step technique do so simply because it takes less time. "I own my own dance studio, and if I don't work I don't get paid," says Suzanne. "If it weren't for the single-stage option, I don't know if I would have had the surgery at all. I knew about the other more drawn-out processes, but I really needed to get it over with and have minimal recovery time. It turned out I was back teaching two weeks after my surgery."

However, it's important to note that just because these newer techniques are considered "one stage" because the mastectomy and implant reconstruction are done at the same time, that doesn't mean you won't have more than one surgery. "It's true that you can wake up from the surgery and be finished, but some women do come back for revisions and size or shape adjustments down the road," says Andrew Salzberg, M.D., chief of plastic surgery at Westchester Medical Center in New York, who pioneered the use of AlloDerm in breast reconstruction. Rori, for instance, had the AlloDerm surgery (commonly known as "AlloDerm One Step") but two years later went back to replace her implant because she wasn't happy with some irregularities and rippling. "I was very upset that I had to go back for another operation and deal with the whole recovery process again," she says. "I just figured if I was going through all of this in the first place, I might as well have beautiful breasts. I didn't want to have any regrets. Now I'm happy I had the follow-up surgery because my breasts look so much better. But it definitely wasn't easy."

TISSUE FLAPS

With flap surgeries, tissue is taken either from the abdomen, buttocks, or back to re-create the breasts. Your doctor will help you decide whether you have enough fat tissue to create new breasts. If you choose to have a flap surgery, you're going to hear a lot of odd-sounding options. For instance, the TRAM, Free TRAM, DIEP, and SIEA all take tissue from the abdomen; the SGAP and the IGAP take tissue from the buttocks; and the LAT flap takes tissue from the back. The difference between each comes down to technique—some involve **microsurgery**, which means the surgeon detaches the tissue, removes it, and then reattaches it to veins and arteries in the breast. With others, like the TRAM and LAT flap, the surgeon tunnels the tissue from the donor site to the breasts without ever removing it. Again, your doctor can explain which techniques are available and might be right for you.

Pros of Implants
- The surgery can take half the time of a flap surgery and require a shorter hospital stay. And the shorter the surgery, the fewer the surgical risks.

- This procedure involves only one initial surgery and one scar site.
- Less anesthesia is used and there's often less pain.
- Breasts won't sag over time (many women don't have to wear bras and just wear adhesives called "petals" to prevent their nipples from protruding).

Cons of Implants
- When there's a foreign object in the body, the body isolates it by creating scar tissue around it. That scar tissue is called a capsule. Sometimes women with implants experience capsular contraction, where the capsule thickens and tightens to the point that it can cause the breast to become hard, misshapen, and in some cases, very painful. A doctor might need to surgically remove the extra tissue.
- Implants can leak or rupture. When saline ruptures, the body absorbs the saline and often the breast deflates immediately. When silicone ruptures, the implant is contained within the breast capsule, so it's not always obvious. Those women might experience asymmetry or hardness, and might need an ultrasound or MRI to determine if the implant is still intact.
- Implants are not considered "lifetime" devices. According to the manufacturers, many implants will have to be replaced at some point.

Pros of Flap Surgery
- The flap is fully integrated into your body—it completely becomes a part of you. So, if you gain or lose weight, your breasts will, too.
- There's no foreign substance in your body.

- This procedure can help get rid of unwanted fat tissue in the area from where you remove the fat, such as your stomach or buttocks.
- Because doctors are using a patient's own tissue, the new breasts will likely have a more natural look and feel than implants would.

Cons of Flap Surgery

- These operations leave two surgical sites and scars, both from where the tissue was taken and on the breast.
- There can also be complications at the donor sites, such as abdominal hernias, muscle damage or weakness, and infections.
- During the surgery, the flap tissue can die (a condition called necrosis). If that happens, the surgeon will either have to try a flap from another part of the body or put in implants.
- Flap surgery can take at least twice as long as an implant surgery, which can increase the odds of surgical complications. It also entails a longer hospital stay.

Re-creating the Nipple and Areola

For women who undergo reconstruction but don't have nipple-sparing procedures, some opt to reconstruct their nipples at some point. Oftentimes, a surgeon will want to wait until any swelling has gone down and the patient is happy with the results, so that he re-creates the nipple and areola in the correct spot. There are countless ways this can be done. For instance, some doctors will take a flap of skin from another part of the body—such as the inner thigh—to make the nipple. Others will fold and tuck the breast skin origami-style to re-create it. Then the surgeon or another health professional may tattoo the areola to reproduce pigment in the skin. This process is usually painless, as the reconstructed areola will typically have little, if any, sensation.

surgical options for ovarian cancer risk

OOPHORECTOMY

For women with a BRCA mutation, their best bet for reducing the odds of getting ovarian cancer is by having an oophorectomy (surgical removal of the ovaries). This operation reduces these women's chances of getting breast cancer by approximately 50 percent and their chances of getting ovarian cancer by about 80 percent, according to a report in the *Journal of the National Cancer Institute* that was a comprehensive analysis of ten previous studies involving BRCA carriers who had already had the surgery. Doctors usually remove the fallopian tubes, too, since women with a hereditary risk of breast and ovarian cancer have an increased risk of developing tubal cancer as well. This kind of surgery is called a bilateral salpingo-oophorectomy, and though it reduces ovarian cancer risk more than any other option, it doesn't eliminate all of it. "There is some residual risk because cancer may start in the peritoneal lining," explains Andrew Berchuck, M.D., director of gynecologic oncology at Duke University Medical Center in North Carolina. (This is called peritoneal cancer, which differs from ovarian cancer in origin but is treated as if it were ovarian cancer.)

While an oophorectomy has obvious benefits, it destroys fertility and can increase a woman's odds of osteoporosis, and heart disease. And it also puts a woman into early menopause, which, for many who have already had children, is the main reason for putting this surgery off. When she first found out the extent of her risk, Rori just wasn't ready to have her ovaries removed. "I was so terrified of aging before my time and removing the parts of my body which keep women vivacious and young," she says. But that changed as she approached forty. "The older I got, the more I started worrying about ovarian cancer,"

Rori says. "My mother had died from the disease and my sister had just battled it. My CA-125 levels were elevated, and I had already had so many close calls with my cysts. I felt more and more that my ovaries were a ticking time bomb. Plus, I had my three kids and didn't want any more. I knew it was time to go ahead with the surgery." So at age thirty-eight, Rori had a bilateral salpingo-oophorectomy. And she says that while she originally had hot flashes, fatigue, vaginal dryness, and a decrease in sex drive, she got her symptoms under control after trying different hormonal replacement options and, she says, by living a healthy lifestyle.

Suzanne and Amy both have BRCA mutations and know that, eventually, they will have their ovaries removed. But they're just not ready. Suzanne says she doesn't want to deal with the potential symptoms of menopause such as wrinkles, exhaustion, and especially weight gain. "I'm a dance teacher who was never naturally thin, and I've had to battle my weight my whole life," she says. "I'd be lying if I didn't admit that that's a big factor on my mind. Maybe if there were confirmed cases of ovarian cancer in my family, like Rori had, I'd be more willing to have the surgery sooner. For now, I'll do surveillance, take birth control pills, and put this surgery off until I'm ready." Adds Amy, who recently got divorced, "I know I should have had my ovaries removed by now, but I feel like I have so much going on with my family and three kids. It's just not a good time. I know that's not an excuse, and I want to get this surgery over with. I hopefully will have it sooner than later."

HYSTERECTOMY

Along with an oophorectomy, some women, like Rori, opt to also have a hysterectomy—the surgical removal of their uterus. If you keep your uterus, you're still at risk for uterine cancer. Plus, even if you have your fallopian tubes removed along with the ovaries, a small bit is still attached to the uterus. Theoretically, that portion of the fallopian tubes could also develop into cancer. However, a hysterectomy may lead to diminished sexual function and bladder problems, especially, some experts say, if your cervix is removed along with your uterus (this is called a total hysterectomy). It's important that, with the help of your doctor, you weigh the risks of the surgery with the potential benefits. In Rori's case, after talking with her gynecologist she decided to have a subtotal hysterectomy, which removes just the upper part of the uterus, but not the cervix.

HOW THE SURGERIES ARE PERFORMED

Traditionally, oophorectomies and hysterectomies were performed by **laparotomy**, an incision across the stomach, which required several days' stay in the hospital. This procedure, performed under general anesthesia, can lead to infection, bleeding, and damage to other organs. While doctors still perform laparotomies, there are now minimally invasive procedures available as well. **Laparoscopy** puts a scope through the belly button, allowing the doctor to see the ovaries. It can be done as an outpatient and involves smaller incisions and a shorter recovery time than a laparotomy. Plus, the cosmetic outcome tends to be better. A much more recent development in technology is a laparoscopic variation called **robotic surgery**. With this minimally invasive option, a robot holds the surgical instruments while the surgeon looks at a three-dimensional image of the patient and manipulates the robot to perform the surgery. Experts say that robotic surgery offers clinical benefits equal to traditional laparoscopic surgery, and it also involves less bleeding, fewer complications, and a quicker recovery.

making a choice

When it comes to deciding how to tackle your risk, there's no right or wrong answer. While medical experts, family, and friends might give you their opinions, ultimately it's your choice and no one should tell you what to do or when. "It took me a long time to absorb the shock of having a genetic mutation and gaining the strength to deal with it," says Amy. "But finally, after nine months of doing research on my different options, I was ready to take that next step. I decided that I wanted to remove as much of my risk as possible by having a bilateral prophylactic mastectomy."

In fact, Lisa, Mayde, Amy, Rori, and Suzanne all chose to have total nipple-sparing mastectomies with silicone implants—specifically AlloDerm-assisted reconstruction with the same team of doctors in New York. That surgery is actually the common denominator that brought the five of them together. However, while Suzanne decided she wanted to have a mastectomy, saw Mayde's results and thought, "I'll take that," most people's decision processes are a lot more drawn out, and often continually evolving.

Mayde, for one, had chosen surveillance for nearly twenty years. But when she had that last MRI that showed her cells were proliferating further toward breast cancer, that was the final straw. "When I got those results, I knew I wanted my breast tissue out," she says. "While I was doing all of my research, I posted on a message board on FORCE and said, 'Has anyone out there had a one-stage procedure?' This woman named Sharon said she had just had one, and the doctor had used a material called AlloDerm. I called her and after learning more about this operation, it sounded like exactly what I was looking for. I then found out that Sharon's breast surgeon was Roy Ashikari, the surgeon my mother saw twenty-five years earlier who had warned me to be careful. That was it! I had found my answer. It was such a relief. I had agonized for so long, but I finally figured out what I was going to do."

Rori in particular said making a decision was very complicated and confusing. "For a long time, I was opposed to the idea of having a prophylactic mastectomy because I thought it was extreme for someone who didn't have cancer to have this surgery," she says. "My breasts were so important to me—I breast-fed my kids with them and they were a huge part of my sexuality. Plus, because I had already had an oophorectomy, my risk of breast cancer was lowered. I was ahead of the game." However, one year after her oophorectomy, Rori had to have a biopsy for a suspicious lump in her breast. Then, a week later, she had to have a second biopsy on the same lump because doctors wanted to examine it further. And even though the lump turned out to be benign, Rori started to change her mind about having a mastectomy. "Going through those biopsies and dealing with the stress of waiting to hear the results was too much for me," she says. "I always felt that, because of my family history, ovarian cancer was what I had to worry about, but these biopsies seemed to be a warning sign that breast cancer could get me, too." Rori started to research her options. At first, she was wary of having any kind of mastectomy, but when she learned about nipple-sparing procedures she realized she could go through with one. "I figured as long as my breasts were mine on the outside, I didn't care what was on the inside," she says.

Lisa also had a lot of trouble rationalizing her choice to have a mastectomy, mostly because her risk wasn't nearly as high as that of other women having the surgery. "I couldn't help thinking, 'I'm BRCA-negative. Am I overreacting?'" Lisa says. "When I met with a breast surgeon to discuss the surgery, he sat me down and said, 'You're in a gray zone. Because your risk isn't as high as someone with, say, a BRCA gene mutation, it's not medically indicated that you have this surgery.' He added, 'I understand why you want to have it, and it's your choice. But don't rush into anything. Think things through.' I followed his advice and booked the surgery for three months out rather than right away so that I'd have plenty of time to cancel it. For those three months I agonized over it and changed my mind a thousand times. It was particularly difficult to go through all this without my mother. She and I always talked extensively about big decisions, and I really wished she had been there to help me make this one. In my heart, I know she would have wanted me to have the surgery. She would have said, 'Just do it and be rid of this risk.' In the end, I felt the same way—I was sick of living in fear. I wanted to move on with my life."

Keep in mind that two women with the exact same risk might choose a very different course of action based on their own personal experiences. For instance, some women might be wary of chemo-prevention or prophylactic surgery because of potential side effects. Others, like the women in this book, are willing to do anything to reduce their risk of breast cancer because they've witnessed loved ones suffer from the disease and, in some cases, die from it. Ultimately, it comes down to learning about your options, getting opinions from experts, and figuring out how and when you want to tackle your risk. "Throughout this whole process, I always felt like some doctors were advising me as though I had cancer growing in my body," Rori says. "I was thinking, 'Slow down. I don't have cancer. I am not sick!' I needed to make my decision on my own terms in my own time frame—that's the only way I could know I made the right one for me."

money matters

Once you've decided on surveillance or an option to lower your risk for breast cancer, the next step is usually to figure out "What will this cost?" and "Will insurance cover it?" Of course, the answers to these questions are often not black and white. "There are so many variables that determine what people will wind up paying for medical services," says Nancy Davenport-Ennis, CEO and founder of the Patient Advocate Foundation. "Each medical provider establishes what [it is] going to charge, and then insurers determine what they are going to reimburse. Also, cost greatly depends on the specific features of your insurance plan. For these reasons, there's no uniformity of prices."

Amy says she felt like it was a full-time job figuring out the costs related to her genetic testing, surveillance, and prophylactic mastectomy. "Those financial aspects were so complicated and confusing, and they added so much anxiety to an already stressful situation," she says. "Like a lot of people, I was always in the dark about what I'd wind up paying out of pocket. I learned that you really have to be your own advocate when dealing with the costs of health care, but it's certainly not simple."

This chapter will help guide you through these financial issues. But keep in mind that prices will vary greatly based on your specific medical needs, your insurance coverage (if any), which doctor you choose, and which city and state you live in. Before you go ahead with any kind of counseling, testing, surveillance, or preventative measures, talk to your doctors and their office managers to find out exactly what costs you might incur.

cost confusion

When it comes to health care in the United States, people often have no idea what they'll wind up paying for a particular treatment or operation. It's not like when you go to the grocery store and you know you'll owe $3.50 for a gallon of milk because it says so on the carton. There's no price list saying how much genetic counseling, a mammogram, MRI, or prophylactic mastectomy costs—expenses will differ from person to person. It's not uncommon for a patient in, say, New York, to pay four times the amount another patient might pay for the same procedure in Iowa. And even if you know how much a doctor might charge for a surgery, for example, keep in mind that those fees don't include bills from hospitals and anesthesiologists, which can add thousands or even tens of thousands of dollars to the overall cost.

Also, many women say that even when they do get their bills, they're still confused as to whether or not they're correct. "When I got my invoices from the hospital after my mastectomy, there were all these charges for 'miscellaneous' items," says Amy. "I had no idea what 'miscellaneous' was referring to, but I wound up just paying the bill because I really didn't even think to question it. I now realize that I should have questioned everything. For instance, I didn't ask, 'How much is it?' every time I took a pill when I was in the hospital, but in retrospect, I should have."

Rori learned the importance of keeping track of costs when she was managing finances for her mother, who was battling ovarian cancer at the time. "That's when I realized that you really have to look over your bills with a fine-toothed comb because they're often filled with mistakes," says Rori. In fact, when Rori had to have a revision surgery a few years after her mastectomy, she was under the impression that her insurance company would pay for it in full. So she was shocked when she got two bills from her doctor's office totaling $16,000. "I called the office and said nicely, 'Excuse me, but I already paid for my initial surgery. I would like to know why I'm getting a bill for $16,000,'" recalls Rori. "The officer manager put me on hold. A few minutes later, she came back on the line and said, 'I'm so sorry. That was a mistake. We really apologize. Just disregard the bill.'"

While that example might be extreme, Rori says that many times she's been billed for something her insurance is covering or she's received two bills for the same treatment. Luckily she keeps on top of it. "Before I write any checks, I wait to see what my insurance has taken care of so I know exactly what I'll owe out of pocket. I keep a log of what I've paid and the status of any bill I've had a problem with. If I immediately wrote a check for any bill I received, there would have been many times that I would have overpaid. It would have taken forever to get that money back—if I got it back at all."

A key to managing health care finances is working with your doctors to understand how much you'll be paying for any procedure, test, or office visit *before* it takes place. Amy says that not doing that was one of the biggest mistakes she made. She says, "One of the doctor's offices once told me, 'You have a $2,000 deductible, of which you have met $336. Then you are covered at 60 percent with a max out of pocket of $8,000. We will collect your remaining deductible up front and then bill your co-insurance of 60 percent after surgery.' This was so baffling to me. Based on this information, I still had no idea how much I'd wind up paying. I was covered at 60 percent, but 60 percent of what?" The key is to ask as many questions as possible until you have a clear idea of what fees you will face. Also, don't be shy about negotiating such prices with your doctors or, if you can't afford one lump sum, asking if they can work out a payment plan.

Just to give you an idea of what different options might cost if you completely paid out of pocket, below is a rough estimate. Again, these prices do *not* take into account hospital, anesthesia or pathology costs, or what insurance companies might cover. For the surgical procedures, there's a great range—the low end indicates Medicare reimbursement rates, but for non-Medicare patients most doctors will charge much more. And for *all* of these costs, prices are subject to change.

TYPICAL COSTS

Genetic counseling session: About $100 to $200 per session. (Most women usually have one or two sessions.)

Genetic testing: The cost of a BRACAnalysis test is between $440 and $3,120, depending on whether you're testing for a founder mutation or a single-site mutation, or you're getting a full-sequencing test (see Chapter 4).

Screening mammogram: $80 to $150

Screening digital mammogram: $130 to $250

Breast ultrasound: $80 to $175

Breast MRI: $850 to $2,000

Raloxifene: The average cost of a month's supply of the brand Evista is about $125. (The generic of raloxifene is not yet available.)

Tamoxifen: The average cost of a month's supply of generic tamoxifen is about $40, depending on the dosage. (The brand name Nolvadex is no longer being manufactured in the United States, though you still might be able to order it through your pharmacy. However, it will cost two to three times more than the generic.)

Bilateral prophylactic mastectomy: About $1,500 to $8,000 or higher (prices vary greatly, depending which procedure you choose).

Reconstruction: $2,500 to $25,000 or higher (prices vary greatly, depending on which procedure you choose).

Nipple reconstruction: Between $1,200 and $6,000 (includes both sides).

Nipple tattooing: About $1,000 or less (includes both sides).

Oophorectomy: $1,000 or higher (prices can vary, based on whether you choose a laparotomy or laparoscopic surgery).

Oophorectomy with hysterectomy: $1,500 or higher.

insurance issues

No one ever said dealing with insurance companies was easy. In some cases it can be a nightmare—Suzanne, for one, knows of a woman whose insurance was denied for some reason while she was lying on the operating table in the hospital, about to get anesthesia before her mastectomy. On the other hand, most women wouldn't be able to consider any means of fighting their breast cancer risk if weren't for health insurance. "I feel lucky that my insurance company did the right thing by me," says Lisa. "If my MRIs and my surgery weren't covered, I wouldn't have been able to go through with them."

When it comes to fighting risk, there are different insurance issues to face each step of the way. For starters, not all insurance companies will cover genetic counseling, though an increasing number of insurers *are* starting to understand its importance, says Angela Trepanier, past president of the National Society of Genetic Counselors. "We're moving in the direction where we'll have uniform coverage of these services," she adds. For instance, some major health insurance providers are starting to cover over-the-phone genetic counseling to their customers. As for genetic testing, Myriad, the sole provider of the BRACAnalysis test, has a reimbursement assistance program that can help you determine if your health insurance company will cover it (call 1-800-469-7423). Most insurers will, but some won't. This program can also help you get preauthorization coverage for genetic testing, and it will help you fight any denials.

Coverage for increased surveillance is also not completely clear-cut. Most insurance plans will cover a yearly mammogram, according to the American College of Radiology. Many do not cover breast MRIs, though some are beginning to do so for high-risk women. As for chemoprevention options, some insurers will cover tamoxifen and raloxifene, others will not. Coverage also depends on whether your specific benefits include prescription drugs.

For women who opt to have a prophylactic mastectomy, the good news is that the Women's Health and Cancer Rights Act of 1998 requires health plans that cover mastectomies to also pay for prostheses, breast reconstruction, and treatment for any physical complications due to the surgery. Despite the name of the act, it does not apply only to cancer patients—women having a prophylactic mastectomy are entitled to the same benefits. However, when it comes to choosing what kind of reconstruction you'd like to have, check with your insurance company to see if they will approve that particular technique. They're only required to pay for options covered in their plan (for instance, not all companies will cover some newer procedures). Also, certain church and government plans may not be required to pay for reconstructive surgery at all. If you are insured under either, check with your plan administrator to see if you're covered.

Again, when it comes to insurance companies, there's no uniformity of coverage, so it's impossible to say what you might wind up paying. Some plans might cover most if not all of your costs, while others won't cover much at all. That's why it's important to make sure you understand your plan ahead of time, so you don't wind up with a bill you can't afford.

first steps

Lisa knew that when dealing with her insurance company, she had to be prepared. "I didn't have a BRCA gene mutation, which I figured would make it that much harder to get approved for my MRIs and any preventative options," she says. "So when it came time to get preauthorization, I walked into my doctors' offices with every bit of information I could find related to my health for the previous ten years. I included my doctor's notes about my biopsies, sonogram and mammogram films and reports, details about my mother's medical history, and basically whatever was on file." It turned out that Lisa was approved in each case without question.

Here are some tips for getting preauthorization and coverage for medical services:

Get Organized

You can never be too organized when it comes to dealing with insurance companies. Nancy Davenport-Ennis, CEO of the Patient Advocate Foundation, suggests maintaining a notebook in which you can keep track of everyone you talk to about your health insurance issues. For every conversation, write down the date and the name, title, and contact information of the person you spoke with. Ideally, find a notebook with pockets in which you can keep copies of every letter you've sent to your doctors or insurance company and copies of those you've received. Also, keep a paper trail of all correspondence. For example, if your insurer says, 'We'll send the preauthorization letter to you next Monday,' send them an e-mail restating what they've said and ask them to confirm what you've written, suggests Davenport-Ennis. When they do, print the e-mail and save it.

Understand Your Plan

Make sure you have a copy of your health plan and that you know what your deductible, co-payment, and maximum out-of-pocket payments are. If you need help comprehending this information, ask an expert who can review your benefits with you (such as someone in human resources at your place of employment, the business manager at your doctor's office, or a nonprofit organization like the Patient Advocate Foundation). Look for specific language in the plan that the insurance company might use to deny your service. For instance, the plan might include a sentence that says they won't allow an experimental or off-label procedure if it's not for therapeutic intent. If you see that kind of language, your doctor needs to specifically build a strong argument explaining why the procedure *is* necessary. Also, beware of balance bills. If you're using an in-network doctor, your doctor or hospital *cannot* bill you the difference between what they charge for a service and what the insurance company is willing to pay. Most state laws and, in the case of Medicare/Medicaid, federal law prohibits balance billing.

Educate Yourself

Try to learn as much as you can about your risk for breast cancer and the test, chemopreventive drug, or procedure you're hoping to get. The more informed you are, the better prepared you'll be to state your case and, if necessary, fight the insurance company. For instance, it couldn't hurt to find out the costs of having surgery and compare that with what you'd spend on future screening tests, biopsies, and possible treatment for breast cancer. This homework can help you explain to the insurance company that having a preventative mastectomy will only lower *their* costs in the long run. Don't hesitate to ask your doctors or nurses any questions you might have. For more information, you can also check out reliable sources online such as the National Comprehensive Cancer Network (www .nccn.org) and the American Cancer Society (www.acs.org).

Ask for Help

Your medical team can arm you with the information you might need to battle insurance companies. The office managers or surgical coordinators at your doctors' offices or the hospital can often help you the most because they deal with insurance companies all the time.

File Immediately

Submitting claims on time is crucial in terms of receiving reimbursement, so make sure you or your doctor's office file them within the time limits set by your insurance company. Claims filed too late could lead to your having to pay for something that should have been paid by the insurance company. As for preauthorization, make sure you allow enough time to complete the approval process when scheduling your test or surgery. In other words, you don't want to schedule, say, an MRI, without leaving time to make sure it's covered *beforehand*.

handling denials

A few weeks before her surgery, Suzanne received distressing news. Though one week earlier her insurance company had sent her an approval letter for a prophylactic mastectomy with doctors in New York, the company then decided to reverse their decision. Her request was denied. "I was shocked," recalls Suzanne. "As soon as I got the initial approval letter, I had scheduled my surgery, booked hotel and airfare, and made arrangements to miss work. My sister also made plans to fly from New Mexico to Florida to help take care of my daughter, Nina, while I was gone. So when my primary care physician called to tell me my insurer had overturned the approval, I was devastated. I had made all these plans never thinking in a million years that they could then deny my mastectomy. My whole world was turned upside down.

"I called up my insurance company and said, 'I have this letter saying my surgery was approved. I've already made my appointment and bought plane tickets. You're going to have to let me go now,'" Suzanne recalls.

"The woman on the line said, 'No. We're not going to be able to do that.'

"But this can't be possible. I have it in writing!

"The woman responded curtly, 'Yes, actually we can overturn our decisions. It is possible.'

"What the hell could I do?" Suzanne adds. "I knew I was in for a fight."

Unfortunately, when it comes to dealing with insurance companies, denials are often part of the game. But it's important to keep in mind that it's not the end of the line if you're denied. In fact, according to a report by the Patient Advocate Foundation, about half of all health claim denials are overturned during the appeals process.

Here are some tips on how to fight denials:

Understand Why You're Denied

If you don't have a copy of the denial in writing, immediately request one. The letter should include the specific reason for the denial. Sometimes the issue can be a simple mistake, such as one misplaced digit in the billing code. Other times, it's not the procedure itself being denied, but an out-of-network doctor. In other words, you can't put up a fight unless you know exactly what it is that you're fighting. In Suzanne's case, her HMO denied what they considered to be off-label use of AlloDerm, the acellular material that would make her direct-to-implant procedure possible.

Gather More Information

"When we issue a denial, a majority of the time, we don't have all the facts," explains Douglas Hadley, M.D., medical officer for CIGNA, a leading health care insurance and service company. In fact, additional information that proves medical necessity is the most common reason for a denial being overturned. Make sure your physician provides the insurance company with a letter addressing the efficacy of the procedure, medication, or test you'd like to get, along with scientific evidence that it's effective and indicated for *you*. You can find such studies by doing a search on www.pubmed.gov. Also, if you have a BRCA gene mutation, you may also want to ask a genetics expert to write a letter explaining your risk statistics. Last, national organizations such as the National Comprehensive Cancer Network and the American Cancer Society set guidelines for who should consider genetic counseling, testing, increased surveillance, and preventative measures. Insurance companies often follow such guidelines, so send a copy of them along with your appeal.

Get Personal, but Keep Your Emotions in Check

The best appeals are often ones that include complete medical records as well as a concise letter from the patient (and/or their prescribing doctor) about their personal and family history. However, says Nancy Davenport-Ennis, don't become too emotional. "Some people are so distraught during the appeals process that they file an appeal expressing all of their feelings," she says. "Remember that, to the health plan, this is nothing but a contract dispute." Instead, explain why you think their decision was wrong and what specific part of your plan supports why you should be covered. Also, add any information, such as details about a strong family history of breast cancer, that would support this intervention. For more help on writing an appeals letter, the Patient Advocate Foundation offers a detailed guide (www.patientadvocate.org).

Start the Appeals Process

Whether you or your doctor's office handles the appeal, you should work closely with your medical team every step of the way. Sometimes it might take three separate appeals to get approval. Typically, the first two sets of appeals are handled internally—medical officers from the insurance company will evaluate your claim. The third appeal might be internal or external, which means a panel of medical specialists not affiliated with the insurance company is called in to review the case. If you're denied three times, the next course of action is to determine your type of policy. If it is self-funded, which means that the employer determines benefit coverage, you may have the option for a "compassionate exception." In these cases, you'd write a compelling letter explaining why you need a particular service in hopes that the employer will overlook contractual language and overturn the appeal. If that doesn't work, or if your plan is not self-funded, then your only other recourse is legal intervention through the court system.

Read the Fine Print

It might sound obvious, but make sure you follow instructions when you file your appeal. Check for any condition of approvals and find out exactly how your insurance company wants you to send the appeal (i.e., Do they want an electronic copy? To whom should you address it?). Most important, note that many insurers have a time limit for you to file an appeal (often sixty days). If you miss the deadline, you might forfeit your right to do so.

Don't Give Up

Suzanne understands the value of persistence all too well. "After my surgery was denied, I was livid, yelling at anyone at my insurance company I could get on the phone," she says. "I kept asking how they could take back their approval. How could they do this to me? Maybe they think people will take no for an answer, but I just kept fighting.

"My insurer would have covered traditional surgery with expanders, but I really needed to have a surgery with the quickest recovery time possible," Suzanne adds. "At the time, my best option was the surgery that used AlloDerm."

Suzanne enlisted some help, and her story is a good example of why it's so important to find a good medical team (as detailed in Chapter 9). "Beth, the surgical coordinator at my plastic surgeon's office, took the bull by the horns," Suzanne recalls. "She said, 'This happens all the time. Don't worry about it. We'll take care of it.' Beth arranged a conference call between my doctor, a representative from the manufacturers of AlloDerm, and the chief medical officer at my insurance company. Four days later, Beth called me and said that my surgery had been reapproved.

"I was so relieved," says Suzanne. "Here I was all geared up to have this surgery, and I didn't want to delay it any longer. I had rearranged my whole schedule for the operation, and I didn't know when I'd be able to do that again. And even though I only wound up paying $150 for the mastectomy along with hotel and airfare, I'm still angry. I keep thinking, 'What about people who aren't approved, especially those who have cancer? I had time and energy to deal with insurance because I was healthy. But what if I had a tumor in my breast?'"

genetic discrimination

Dealing with insurance companies is tricky enough, which is why many people are reluctant to get tested for the BRCA gene mutations. They figure if they have one, they don't want to have to disclose that information to insurance companies or employers. "When my doctor told me not to get tested because I'd 'never get health insurance again' if I were positive, that became my reason for not getting tested for nearly thirteen years, until I learned that he was wrong," says Suzanne. Other women who choose to get genetic testing opt to pay out of pocket because of the fear of such potential discrimination. "When I got tested, it was relatively new and very hush-hush," says Rori. "I thought that from the insurance company's perspective, testing positive for BRCA would be as bad as being sick with some horrible disease. I didn't want to take a chance, so I paid for the test out of pocket." Then, when Rori did test positive, she made sure she reminded her physicians to avoid writing "BRCA1" in her records on every visit. Instead, they'd just used the words "high risk."

Truth be told, however, there are very few accounts of genetic discrimination in insurance companies ever happening. Plus, there are laws in place protecting consumers, the most important one being the Genetic Information Nondiscrimination Act (GINA), which became effective in 2009. This act prohibits insurers from using genetic information to deny benefits or raise premiums for both group and individual policies. It also prevents employers from collecting genetic information or using it to make decisions about hiring, firing, or compensation. "Most people don't have to fear discrimination anymore because insurance companies can't require people to disclose that information and, even if they do find out about it, they can't use the information to make enrollment or coverage decisions," says Joann Boughman, Ph.D. executive vice president of the American Society of Human Genetics. In other words, even if you list a BRCA mutation as a preexisting condition, insurance companies can't penalize you.

However, when it comes to employer discrimination, GINA does not apply to companies with fourteen or fewer people or to people in the military. "Theoretically, if a small employer found out someone was BRCA-positive, they could fire that person without any repercussions under the federal GINA legislation," says Dr. Boughman. Also, GINA (or any federal laws for that matter) does not protect against genetic discrimination in regards to life insurance. If you're interested in purchasing a life insurance policy, experts recommend you do so before going through with genetic testing.

Strides are being made against genetic discrimination, but we have a long way to go. With GINA, there's one less barrier, but many people still remain skeptical. Lisa, for example, has a friend whose mother died of ovarian cancer. She clearly has a reason to test, but says she's afraid to because of discrimination. "I told her it's not like that, but she doesn't believe me," says Lisa. "I hear it from people all the time— they're afraid they won't get health insurance if they have a genetic mutation so they avoid the test altogether. Their mentality is that they'll have a strike against them. They'll be labeled. It might not be the case, but that's how people feel."

for the uninsured

One of Mayde's closest friends, Jane, is uninsured. She's self-employed and just couldn't afford the $600 a month she was paying for insurance, so she gave it up. What worries Mayde is that her friend's mother battled breast cancer and eventually died of brain cancer. Some of Jane's other family members have battled cancer as well. But she won't do anything about her own risk.

"One day, Jane told me she hasn't had a mammogram in two years and has never had a breast MRI," says Mayde.

"I asked her, 'What are you doing? You have to keep on top of these things.'

"Jane said, 'I can't afford to have a mammogram. I had to drop my insurance. What can I do?'

"It makes me sad hearing about women who do nothing about their breast cancer risk because of cost," says Mayde. "I feel like they're forced to play Russian roulette with their lives. For a woman who develops breast cancer, skipping even one yearly mammogram can make such an enormous difference in her prognosis."

The truth is, there *are* options for women who are underinsured or uninsured. These include:

National Breast and Cervical Cancer Early Detection Program

This program provides breast and cervical cancer early detection testing to low-income women without health insurance for free or at a low cost. Such services include clinical breast exams, mammograms, pelvic exams, and pap smears. The program also provides diagnostic testing and surgical consultation. To learn more about it, contact 800-232-4636. Or check out www.cdc.gov/cancer/nbccedp.

Susan G. Komen for the Cure

This organization offers educational and support resources for breast cancer and grants funds to organizations and programs throughout the country that offer aid ranging from free or low-cost mammograms to chemoprevention. To find such services in your area, visit www.komen.org or call Susan G. Komen for the Cure's breast care helpline at 877-GO-KOMEN.

Myriad Genetic Laboratories, Inc.

Myriad (the sole provider of the BRACAnalysis test) offers free genetic testing to uninsured patients who meet certain medical and financial criteria (www.myriadtests.com).

Partnership for Prescription Assistance (PPA)

Sponsored by the Pharmaceutical Research and Manufacturers of America (PhRMA), PPA helps people with a low income and no prescription coverage. This organization provides access to 475 different programs that together provide more than 2,500 different prescription drugs for free or at a very low cost. These drugs include tamoxifen and raloxifene. If you need financial assistance for such prescriptions, call PPA at 888-477-2669 or check out www.pparx.org.

Right Action for Women

Founded by actress Christina Applegate after she was diagnosed with breast cancer, this organization helps high-risk women who don't have the insurance or financial means to cover breast screenings, such as MRIs. (www.rightactionforwomen.org)

Community Programs

Contact your local hospitals to find out if they offer any free or low-cost surveillance. For example, some have mammography vans that drive around to various sites offering mammograms, sometimes at discount costs.

Medicaid

Medicaid is a state-federal partnership program for low-income people who are either disabled, pregnant, children, or older than sixty-five. Call the department of health in your state to find out what options Medicaid will cover and if you meet your state's requirements.

be your own advocate

For some people like Mayde, Rori, and Lisa, dealing with the costs of health care and insurance isn't as dreadful as it seems. "I was worried about getting approval for my mastectomy because, like Lisa, I didn't have a BRCA gene mutation," says Mayde. "But once my pathology reports came back showing I had lobular carcinoma in situ, a major risk factor for breast cancer, I was quickly approved. It's sad, but in some ways I felt fortunate to have that diagnosis because without it I may have had trouble getting preauthorization for my surgery."

However, Suzanne's and Amy's experiences were challenging. As with Suzanne, Amy had trouble getting approval for her prophylactic mastectomy. "When I tried to get preauthorization, my insurer came back saying I was 'in review,'" she says. "They said they needed the last five years' worth of my medical information. All I could think was that I had already made up my mind to have the surgery, and I didn't want to wait any longer. And though I did eventually get approved, I really felt like I was at the insurance company's beck and call."

Each of these five women said they dealt with their finances by relying on medical experts who could help them and, most important, speaking up for themselves. "I always tried to work out arrangements with my doctor's office if a particular treatment or test was too expensive," says Rori. "Maybe I'd pay in increments or see if they could lower my bill if I paid it in full. It's amazing what health professionals can do for you if you just ask."

Ultimately, handling costs and insurance is never easy, but it's a necessary aspect of combating your breast cancer risk. And, as Lisa, Mayde, Amy, Rori, and Suzanne learned, once you pass this hurdle you will likely realize it was well worth any fight.

a controversial decision

Once you've made a decision about how you want to tackle your odds of getting breast cancer, don't be surprised if everyone doesn't agree with the path you choose. From genetic testing and surveillance to chemoprevention and prophylactic surgery, these topics can be polarizing. Many factors can affect a person's opinion regarding how you should deal with your risk. People close to you might give advice based on good intentions—they want you to do what *they* believe is the right thing. Also, a person's experience with cancer comes into play. For instance, someone whose mom caught cancer early, had a lumpectomy, and survived might think preventative surgeries are too drastic, while a person whose mother died from the disease might believe that surveillance is too risky. And then there are people who are fundamentally opposed to certain risk-reducing drugs and surgeries.

After years of surveillance and agonizing over their risk, Lisa, Mayde, Amy, Rori, and Suzanne each chose to have prophylactic mastectomies— probably the most divisive of all the options. "This is such a personal decision, but it seems everyone has something to say about it," says Lisa. "Before and after my operation, I heard from neighbors, people in the gym, moms at my children's school. Some supported me; others tried to talk me out of it. And who knows what the rest were saying behind my back."

It's difficult enough weighing the options without having to face negativity from friends, loved ones, and strangers. However, knowing what to expect can make dealing with naysayers a little easier. Here's an overview of some of the feedback you might encounter, whether you choose surveillance, a prophylactic mastectomy, or other means of lowering your risk.

a "radical" measure

There is no doubt that a prophylactic mastectomy will reduce your chances of getting breast cancer more than any other option out there. However, some experts say losing your breasts is too high a price to pay. "After all the time and money we've spent on breast cancer research, you'd think we would have made enough progress that women wouldn't be removing their breasts to reduce their risk," says Carolina Hinestrosa, executive vice president of the National Breast Cancer Coalition. "We're throwing our hands up and saying the scientific community has nothing better to offer, so let's take this step. I have grave concerns that too many women believe this surgery is the answer."

One issue some experts have is that, with a prophylactic mastectomy, you're removing a woman's healthy tissue with no absolute certainty that she'll develop breast cancer. In other words, just because you have a high risk doesn't mean you'll get the disease. And it's not just cancer-free women making such a decision—many who have cancer in one breast are opting to have both removed (which is called a contralateral prophylactic mastectomy). A study in the *Journal of Clinical Oncology* found that the rate of women having contralateral prophylactic mastectomies increased 150 percent between 1998 and 2003.

Such women, for instance, might have both breasts removed when a lumpectomy in the one with cancer would suffice.

Other experts point out that a mastectomy is not without risks itself—it's a major surgery that comes with the usual complications that can arise with any operation. And some call attention to the fact that studies haven't shown that people who have prophylactic mastectomies will live longer than those who don't.

Along with dissent in the medical community, the decision to have a prophylactic mastectomy can also be quite controversial among loved ones. "My husband, Jonathan, was initially dead-set against the surgery," recalls Mayde. "He's a radiologist and I think he felt like his specialty (or, in other words, increased surveillance) would save me. When I told him I was booking a consultation with a breast surgeon in New York, Jonathan tried to talk me out of it. He then enlisted a team of experts to explain why I was making the wrong decision. I spoke with one leading breast cancer researcher who said he thought it was ridiculous I would even consider surgery when there were other options. Another breast imaging specialist told me I was being hasty. He said that if I continued doing surveillance and wound up getting breast cancer, it would be caught early and there would be no great threat to my life. I said to him, 'But I'll have breast cancer. And even if they catch it early, I don't want to risk one cancerous cell escaping into my body.' He responded abruptly, 'Well then, your mind is already made up. Good-bye and good luck.'"

Rori adds that, at first, even she considered the whole idea of prophylactic surgery over the top. "When I found out I had a BRCA gene mutation, a gynecologic oncologist told me I should consider removing my breasts and ovaries," she recalls. "I thought, 'Why would a healthy person want to do that?'" However, over time, Rori decided she wanted to reduce her risk for breast and ovarian cancer as much as possible. The way to do that was to have both surgeries. Rori's loved ones were completely behind her decision to have an oophorectomy.

"My friends and family actually thought I'd be crazy if I *didn't* have the operation," says Rori. "My mother died of ovarian cancer, my sister battled it, and I had so many other warning signs that I could be next, such as suspicious ovarian cysts and an elevated CA-125 level. Plus, I already had three kids and wasn't having any more." But two years later, when Rori told those same people she was having a mastectomy, they sang a different tune. "My brother was shocked and just couldn't understand why I'd take out healthy tissue," Rori says. "And to this day, one of my closest friends still thinks I jumped the gun. She thought I should wait, because there are always new tests and treatments."

In fact, that's a common argument—the breast cancer field is constantly evolving and researchers are finding better treatments and preventative measures. "The decision to have a mastectomy is final—there's no turning back," says Michael Stefanek, Ph.D, director of the American Cancer Society's Behavioral Research Center. "So if down the road a breakthrough noninvasive option comes out that reduces risk as much as a mastectomy, will a woman who had a preventative surgery regret her decision and let it haunt her the rest of her life? Or what if there's a genetic test that determines exactly who will get breast cancer, so people would know that having the surgery was necessary to prevent an inevitable disease?"

Lisa says that even among people who weren't necessarily against her decision to have a prophylactic mastectomy, many didn't seem to understand that having the surgery was a choice, not a necessity. "When I told some friends and acquaintances I was having a mastectomy, they'd gasp and make this face, like I'd just told them I have cancer," she says. Adds Mayde, "People to this day think I had my surgery because I had breast cancer. They say, 'Oh, I'm so sorry' and I tell them, 'Don't be. I'm not sick. I'm okay.'"

Also, as discussed in Chapter 6, many doctors are still on the fence as to whether or not to choose nipple-sparing. Some experts believe that if you're going to remove breast tissue you might as well get rid of as much as possible. Others argue that preserving the nipple during a prophylactic mastectomy doesn't seem to lead to more cases of cancer; however, doing so can greatly improve the aesthetic outcome for women.

To get an idea of the type of negative discourse surrounding prophylactic mastectomies, just take a look at message boards, blogs, and other online sources. Suzanne said she was shocked by some of the comments she read on one such site. "People were saying that women having prophylactic surgeries were 'insane,' 'paranoid,' and just doing this for attention," she says. "Many said we were butchering ourselves and called the surgery 'self-mutilation.' One post even likened our surgery to a person removing their eyes because everyone in their family had cataracts and went blind when they were old. And then there was the comment that said removing healthy breasts is 'stupid' and a 'slap in the face to women who actually have breast cancer.' I just sat in front of the computer, stunned. The conviction behind some of these comments just blew my mind."

a viable option

While plenty of people might argue that a prophylactic mastectomy is a radical measure, others think it's a worthwhile choice. "No physician envisions building the future of breast cancer prevention on removing breasts," says Patrick Borgen, M.D., a leading breast surgeon and director of the Brooklyn Breast Cancer Program at Maimonides Medical Center in New York. "One day there will be better ways to medically or genetically prevent this disease. The problem is, that day is not here yet. We can't put our heads in the sand and ignore the fact that some women will benefit from prophylactic mastectomies. It's the best weapon we have. Some people say the price is too high, but who are they to say how valuable a woman's breasts are to her, especially when she's buried a mother, sister, or other loved one from the disease?"

Suzanne says she couldn't agree more. "Of course, it's extreme that in order to prevent breast cancer, you have to have a major surgery. But is it overkill? Absolutely not. I saw close relatives suffer through chemotherapy and die horrible, agonizing deaths. I'd do anything to avoid that. To me, having surgery is nothing compared to a battle with cancer."

Part of the reason why more women are considering prophylactic mastectomies than ever before is that the reconstruction options are so much better than they were years ago. Today, with a skin-sparing mastectomy, doctors can leave the appearance of the breast nearly intact and just remove the dangerous tissue inside. Mayde says it seems many people don't realize that having a mastectomy doesn't mean you'll be left flat as a board. "I always hear people saying things like, 'Oh my God, they're cutting breasts off. How horrible.' It might have been like that thirty years ago when a mastectomy meant having the radical, deforming surgery my mother had. But it's not like that anymore. Having the skin-sparing procedure, I don't feel like I lost my breasts at all. In fact, I think they look better than ever."

Another reason women opt to have a double mastectomy is that they figure they're avoiding not only breast cancer itself, but also years of breast screening, possible biopsies, and all of the anxiety that goes along with worrying about the disease. As Dr. Borgen puts it, they're "removing the swords hanging over their heads."

In truth, many women say that eliminating fear is the biggest motivating factor. "I was so terrified that one day I'd wind up with cancer, the courage to have the surgery was less than the courage I needed to sit around and wait for the other shoe to drop," says Suzanne. "Having grown up without a mother, I'd do whatever I could to make sure the same thing didn't happen to my daughter." Adds Amy, "I really think it was inevitable I would have gotten breast cancer, especially considering my aunt, mother, and grandmother all battled the disease. And I figured that if I did get it, I'd probably wind up having a mastectomy anyway. But then I'd also possibly need radiation or chemotherapy, and I'd never have peace of mind because I'd always be worried about a recurrence. By having a mastectomy as a preventive surgery, I had the luxury of being in control and making decisions when I was healthy rather than sick. I'll never know if this surgery was necessary, but it was a chance I was willing to take. The alternative was unthinkable."

As for the idea that there might be a cure in ten years, Lisa says she understands the argument. "I hope researchers *do* find a vaccine you get when you're born and that's the end of it," she says. "But there are women who need to make decisions *now* based on what is available today. And even if we do find a cure in a decade, who's to say I wouldn't have had cancer during that time? For me, living those ten years without stress and fear would be worth anything in the world."

While women choosing this surgery might experience some backlash, they will likely find that many people are extremely supportive. "My friends and family told me I was doing something incredibly brave," says Lisa. "They said they'd do the same thing if they were in my position." Suzanne says that though her brother and sister resisted the idea of her having surgery at first, the minute they learned what it meant to have the BRCA gene mutation, they were completely supportive. "My family knows what's in store for someone with a cancer diagnosis," she says. "They witnessed what happens, so no one was going to say this was drastic." And, though Mayde's husband didn't originally agree with her decision to have the surgery, he ultimately stood by her when he learned her breast cells were changing so much that her cancer risk was increasing dramatically. "Jonathan realized that I had to do what I felt was right for me," she says. "He said, 'Mayde, I'm with you 100 percent.'"

other controversies you might face

Though the concept of prophylactic mastectomy can trigger much debate, other issues related to breast cancer risk carry their own controversies as well. Here's what else you might expect:

Genetic testing: Genetic testing can raise some issues for women who test positive for a BRCA mutation, which can mean other family members have it as well. The concern is if and when to tell them. Angela Trepanier of the National Society of Genetic Counselors recommends talking to close family members *before* you get tested so you can get a sense of how they might react once you get results back. "That way, if you test positive, you can come home and call the people who were on board with your having the test in first place," she suggests. "You might as well start by telling people you can expect some support from." Also, she adds that it's important not to blame yourself for how other family members react to the news. "If you contact relatives to let them know there's a BRCA mutation in the family, you're giving them the information as a gift," says Trepanier. "All you can do is make sure they have resources that can help them. After that, you can't take responsibility if they don't act on that knowledge." Rori, for instance, respects her sister Nancie's decision not to test despite their family's multiple battles with cancer and BRCA status. And regarding Suzanne's male cousins who also haven't gone through with genetic testing, Suzanne says, "I can't force my cousins to take the test. I've given them plenty of information about their risk and even mailed them a copy of my positive BRCA results. It's now up to them to do something about it, and I just hope for their daughters' sakes that they do."

Surveillance: When a woman who has a high risk for breast cancer chooses surveillance over a preventative measure, her doctors and loved ones might argue that she's not doing enough to safeguard herself. In turn, many previvors say they feel an enormous pressure to have a prophylactic mastectomy sooner than later. Rori, for one, says she really believed in doing surveillance for as long as possible, but her doctors continually tried to persuade her to have the surgery. (And because of Rori's strong family history of ovarian cancer and BRCA status, her physicians said there was no question she should have her ovaries removed, too.)

Chemoprevention: Some physicians and women still have a difficult time with the concept of using drugs to prevent breast cancer, experts say. That's particularly the case with tamoxifen, which has a stigma attached to it, as it's also used to treat patients who already have the disease. "Many doctors have felt uncomfortable recommending tamoxifen because it was perceived as a 'cancer medicine,'" says Therese Bevers, M.D., medical director of the Cancer Prevention Center at M. D. Anderson Cancer Center in Houston. "There is also a reluctance by women to initiate chemoprevention, probably because of the side effects and the whole idea of having to take a pill every day even though they're not sick."

Oophorectomy: There is some controversy surrounding removal of the ovaries, but not nearly as much as there is surrounding mastectomies. For one, there are no good screening tools for ovarian cancer, which makes it a deadlier disease than breast cancer. Also, an oophorectomy is a two-for-one deal: among BRCA carriers, the surgery lowers the odds of getting breast cancer by almost 50 percent and ovarian cancer by about 80 percent. Plus, there's the fact that ovaries are internal organs and, unlike a mastectomy, the surgery isn't cosmetic.

One area of dissent regarding oophorectomy is *when* to have it. Many experts recommend that women with BRCA gene mutations have their ovaries removed by the time they are thirty-five or done having children (though that decision should be evaluated on a case-by-case basis). But the thought of losing fertility and entering premature menopause is a lot for most women to bear. Amy said she got some flak from several doctors who told her she should have already had her ovaries removed, but to her, the mastectomy was her priority. "Breast cancer, not ovarian cancer, was in my family, so that's what I've been afraid of my whole life," she says. "I know my logic might not be correct, but that's how I felt." Adds David Cohn, M.D., a gynecologic oncologist at the Ohio State University College of Medicine in Columbus, "It's an individual decision based on what a woman brings to the table. One having the surgery might say, 'I saw my mom die of ovarian cancer and I don't want that to happen to me,' while another might say, 'I'll accept the risk for now so that I can have my family.'"

Another point of contention among experts is whether or not to remove the uterus (in other words, have a hysterectomy) along with the ovaries and fallopian tubes. Theoretically, a bit of the fallopian tube left in the uterus can turn cancerous. Also, women who don't have hysterectomies will have an increased risk of uterine cancer if they ever take chemopreventive drugs. On the flip side, however, having the extra surgery brings its own inherent risk—there is a longer recovery time and more risk of surgical complications. Additionally, some women experience decreased sexual function and bladder problems after their hysterectomy. Again, this is an issue you should address with your doctor.

your body, your choice

After getting over her shock at some of the posts she read online, Suzanne said she stopped reading them. "People's comments were so cavalier," she says. "If they haven't lived my life, how dare they judge me for what I'm doing? Do they know what it's like to grow up without a mother? What if it was their wife, mother, or daughter who had such high odds of getting breast cancer? I'm not judging people who don't have the surgery, so I didn't want to be judged because I did. I think people have to do what is right for them."

That's easier to accomplish when a doctor doesn't heavily influence a woman's decision on how to reduce her risk. "A doctor's role is to empower patients by telling them what all of their options are in a non-judgmental way," says Dr. Patrick Borgen of Maimonides Medical Center in New York. "We shouldn't persuade them or dissuade them." In fact, a study in the *Annals of Surgical Oncology* found that women who regret having had a prophylactic mastectomy, albeit a very small percentage, have one thing in common: they feel that their doctor talked them into having it.

As discussed earlier in this chapter, Rori can relate. "I felt a lot of pressure from some physicians. They said my risk was so high I needed to have a mastectomy and oophorectomy sooner rather than later. But if anything, their treating my risk reduction like an emergency completely turned me off. I just didn't understand the urgency. I needed time to let the news that I had a genetic mutation sink in, get second and third opinions, and do my own research. Only then could I figure out what, if anything, would be the best option for me."

Whether you choose surveillance, chemoprevention, preventative surgery, or even nothing, keep in mind that there will be those who support you and those who may not. But the bottom line is to listen to what people have to say, ask for advice from people you trust, and remember that, ultimately, the only opinion that matters is yours.

defusing the time bomb

A STEP-BY-STEP GUIDE TO PROPHYLACTIC SURGERY

As the first of the five previvors in this book to have a prophylactic mastectomy, Mayde was a source of comfort to each of the others, helping them pack for the hospital and explaining what to expect before, during, and after the surgery. She knew firsthand how crucial her support was to her friends. "When I was getting ready for my operation, a woman named Sharon I had met in an online support group became my lifeline," Mayde recalls. "She had already had the surgery and was available day or night to reassure me and answer all of my questions. I was so scared, but Sharon really allayed a lot of my fears. I decided that someday I would do for others what Sharon had done for me."

Women who know they have a high risk for breast cancer often say they feel like they have a "time bomb" ticking within them. In other words, they think it's just a matter of time before they develop the disease. And to many, having a prophylactic mastectomy (and for women who have a BRCA mutation, a prophylactic oophorectomy) is the only way to "defuse" or stop this metaphorical bomb. However, according to a study conducted through the Cancer Research Network, two-thirds of women who had had a mastectomy wished they had had more information about it beforehand. Specifically, women wanted to know more about the reconstruction options available to them and possible complications such as numbing, scars, and pain. Of course, just like with childbirth, nothing can fully prepare you for what it will be like to go through an operation—whether it be a mastectomy or oophorectomy. But learning a little bit more about it can make the process easier to bear.

"When I first decided to have a mastectomy, I was terrified," says Amy. "I had never had a surgery before and was so nervous about all of the unknowns. Luckily, I met Mayde through FORCE. She is so detail-oriented, and she told me every little thing I might need to know, from what pain meds to ask for and what kind of bras to buy to how I might feel and look after the operation. I was still nervous, but it was a lot less daunting knowing what to anticipate each step of the way."

Here's a guide that will help you do just that if you're thinking of having a prophylactic surgery. First, we'll explore mastectomy; then, for women with a BRCA mutation, oophorectomy.

mastectomy: before the surgery

HOW TO FIND DOCTORS

When you're having a mastectomy, a breast surgeon or surgical oncologist will remove as much breast tissue as possible. Then, if you choose to have reconstruction, a plastic surgeon recreates a new breast with either implants or flap tissue. Here are some suggestions on assembling this team of experts:

STEP ONE: LOCATE POSSIBILITIES

Once you've decided to go ahead with a prophylactic mastectomy, your next and possibly most important step is to find a doctor you trust. A great place to start is with your genetic counselor, says Christy Russell, M.D., spokesperson for the American Cancer Society and co-director of the University of Southern California/Norris Lee Breast Center in Los Angeles. "Many genetic counselors are linked to a well-honed group of surgeons who have expertise working with high-risk patients," she says. You can also ask your gynecologist, family doctor, or even women on message boards for referrals. Ideally, find a multi-disciplinary cancer center that offers genetic testing, screening, preventative treatments such as mastectomies, and even psychological care in the same location. These doctors will be used to working together, which is always a plus.

Here are some great resources that can help you find doctors in your area:

Multidisciplinary Centers

- **National Cancer Institute:** This organization supports at least sixty-five cancer centers renowned for their scientific research and multidisciplinary approach to fighting the disease. You can search for these cancer centers by name, state, or region. (cancercenters.cancer.gov)
- **FORCE:** This nonprofit offers a list of clinics that have a multidisciplinary approach to handling women with a high risk for cancer. There are also links to other sites that can help you find reputable experts for mastectomies, breast reconstruction, and oophorectomies. (www.facingourrisk.org)
- **Association of Community Cancer Centers:** More than 670 medical centers, hospitals, cancer programs, and oncology group practices throughout the United States are members of this organization. By searching for centers in your state, you can find out about each program's facilities, staff, services, and more. (www.accc-cancer.org)

- **National Consortium of Breast Centers:** This organization includes more than eight hundred breast centers, ranging from screening centers to comprehensive cancer centers. You can search for breast centers in your area and then check to make sure they offer the services you're looking for. For example, not all breast centers offer a high-risk program. Start by searching among the two hundred centers that participate in a quality review program. (www.breastcare.org)

Doctors Who Perform Mastectomies

- **American Society of Breast Surgeons:** All members are general surgeons with a demonstrated interest in breast surgery; many focus exclusively in that area. Call 877-992-5470 and the society can provide you with a list of members in your area. (www.breastsurgeons.org)
- **Society of Surgical Oncology:** This organization provides contact information for their 2,300 physician members. You can search by name or location. (www.surgonc.org)

Doctors Who Perform Reconstructive Surgery

- **American Society of Plastic Surgeons:** This organization's members are not only board-certified, but they've also completed specific training in plastic surgery and fulfilled certain medical education requirements. You can search for a doctor by name, procedure, or geographical location. (www.plasticsurgery.org)

STEP TWO: CHECK FOR COMPETENCY

After you've found a few options to consider, it's time to determine which surgeon (or possibly multiple surgeons) is the right one for you. Here are some credentials your doctor should have:

Board certification: When a physician is board-certified in a particular area of expertise, that means he or she has earned a license to practice medicine, completed a required residency, and passed a comprehensive examination. Contact the American Board of Medical Specialties to find out if a doctor is board-certified (www.abms.org or 866-ASK-ABMS).

Experience: Often the more surgeries a physician has performed, the more honed is the physician's technique. You wouldn't want to have, say, a particular flap surgery by a doctor who does only a few per year. If you're seeing a general surgeon, what's most important is that a significant part of the doctor's practice is devoted to breast surgery. Also, for a previvor, it can help to find a doctor who works with women who have cancer or with women who have a high risk for developing the disease.

Hospital credentials: Find out where your surgeon is permitted to practice, and then make sure that the Joint Commission has accredited that facility. Such accreditation means that the organization is committed to continually improving quality of care and patient safety. Go to www.qualitycheck.org where you can search facilities by name, location, type of provider, and types of services. If a health care organization is accredited by the Joint Commission, it will have a Gold Seal of Approval and a quality report by its name.

STEP THREE: START INTERVIEWS

Once you've narrowed down your choices, it's time to find the doctor you're happiest moving forward with based on his or her skill and personality. It's not uncommon for patients to interview several doctors: Mayde actually interviewed four breast surgeons and four plastic surgeons until she felt comfortable making a decision. On the flip side, many women are content after meeting with only one doctor. Regardless of the number of physicians you interview, here are some questions you may want to ask:

General Questions

- How many surgeries of this type do you perform each month? Each year?
- Can I see before-and-after pictures of your previous patients?
- Can I speak with any of your former patients who had the surgery I'm having?
- How much will this procedure cost me? Will my insurance cover it, and will you help me with insurance filing?
- Are there any possible complications I should know about?
- Do you keep surveys about your patients' satisfaction rate?
- What am I going to look like?
- How much discomfort or pain do women typically feel afterward?
- How long will my hospital stay and recovery time be?
- When will I be able to return to normal activities such as driving, lifting weights, running, and intercourse?

Questions for a Breast Surgeon

- Are there any plastic surgeons you work with on a regular basis?
- Have any of your patients developed breast cancer after their prophylactic mastectomies?
- Will you consider newer techniques, such as nipple sparing?

Questions for a Plastic Surgeon

- Are there any new reconstruction options I should know about?
- What is the percentage of infection in the first year?

- What kinds of reconstruction are possible for me?
- What is your flap or implant failure rate?
- Will I have any feeling in my reconstructed breast?
- What are my options if I'm unhappy with my results?
- How many of your patients have to undergo revisions after their initial surgery? (Revisions are additional surgeries that doctors perform when their patients are not satisfied with the original results.)

STEP FOUR: MAKE A DECISION

After researching your options, it's time to choose a surgeon. If you've followed the steps above, you can rest assured that you'll be making a thoughtful decision. Keep in mind that, in some cases, the most skilled surgeon might not be the best one for you. You need to also feel comfortable with your doctor, and you shouldn't dismiss your instincts.

PRE-OP CHECKLISTS

When Lisa was getting ready to pack for the hospital, she found many helpful tips on message boards. Mayde and Amy also gave her advice on how to make her surgery run a little smoother. Lisa's preparation paid off. "I felt so helpless after my mastectomy, but luckily I had what I needed to get me through my immediate recovery," she says. "I know I would have been fine if I didn't prepare at all, but having certain things at the hospital and planning for my return home made the experience a little more comfortable for me."

Below are some suggestions:

What to bring to the hospital:
- **Copies of medical records and your insurance card.** If you have a living will, bring a copy of that, too.

- **A list of phone numbers** of anyone you'll want to contact after the surgery.
- **Sleep aids:** Bring earplugs, an eye mask, a white-noise machine, or music to block out noise and light in your hospital room.
- **Small pillows** to keep your arms elevated in the hospital.
- **A journal:** Some women find it cathartic writing about their experience.
- **Sucking candy** to help with a sore throat from having the breathing tube inserted during the surgery. You also might want to bring **lip balm** for chapped lips.
- **Drain attachments:** Bring large safety pins to attach your drains to your gown or bathrobe. (Drains are tubes attached to the surgical sites that remove excess fluid.) Also, you can attach the drains to a makeshift necklace, such as a ribbon or two shoelaces tied together.
- **Proper clothing:** After a mastectomy, you'll need button-down or zip-up blouses, dresses, sweaters, and sweatshirts because you won't be able to put on anything over your head. Also, you'll have drains, so stick with baggy clothes. And bring slip-on shoes and a lightweight robe that ties in the front.
- **Constipation remedies:** Anesthesia and pain narcotics can lead to constipation, so bring stool softeners or mild laxatives with you in case you need them.
- **Post-op bras:** After your surgery, you'll need to wear special mastectomy bras for a few weeks. If your reconstructed breast size will be 34C, however, that doesn't mean you'll definitely need a 34C bra because you have to factor in room for swelling and the drains. Ask your doctor which size bra you should pick up, but your best bet is to purchase several sizes, keep the tags on, and return the ones you don't use.

What else to prepare ahead of time:

- **Try to book the first surgery of the day**, especially since you can't eat or drink anything after midnight the night before. Usually the earlier the surgery, the less likely there will be delays. Suzanne's surgery was supposed to be at noon but got pushed back until two p.m. She says that those two hours might not seem like a big deal, but to her they were torture. "Because I couldn't have my morning cup of coffee, I had the most excruciating caffeine-withdrawal headache," she says. "Plus, the anxiety at that point was overwhelming."

- **At home, put dishes, glasses, clothes, medicine, and anything else you might need at counter level** so you won't have to reach for them after your surgery. You might also want to unscrew caps on items you use frequently (keeping child safety in mind, of course).

- **Ask for your post-surgery prescriptions ahead of time**, so you'll have them filled and ready to go as soon as you leave the hospital.

- **Make meals and freeze them**, or stock up on microwavable entrees.

- **Pick up some cotton balls and rubbing alcohol** for cleaning your surgical site and drains.

- **Buy a small plastic chair for the shower.** You can rest your foot on it while shaving your legs and avoid bending over.

- **Find a temporary purse.** You won't be able to carry weight on your shoulders for a while, so consider using a handheld clutch or other alternative until you're healed.

- **Request a private room at the hospital.** It depends on availability, and there may be a slight added fee. Lisa paid $75 extra a day, but says it was worth the money for the peace, quiet, and privacy.

BUILDING A NETWORK

While bringing along some or all of the items mentioned in the pre-op checklist might help you get through the surgery, often nothing is as important as having friends or even online acquaintances who have been through the same experience.

When you're preparing for a surgery, remember that there's a sisterhood of women out there who have been through it all before. As the women in this book discovered, these other previvors can really tell you all of the nitty-gritty details about the surgery and recovery process. While a surgeon can tell you about the operation itself, he might not be able to help guide you through the more emotional and psychological issues.

Lisa says that Amy and Mayde helped her every step of the way when it came to her prophylactic mastectomy. "I met with the girls when I was considering my surgery," she says. "They showed me their reconstructed breasts and were instrumental in giving me an idea of what the operation entailed and what I might look like. Then, once I made a decision, I had a tough time coming to terms with it. Talking to the two of them and seeing that they had few regrets really helped me. They also gave me very different perspectives: Mayde kept telling me how easy the surgery was going to be, while Amy explained that everyone's experience is different and that my breasts would never feel the same again. I loved Mayde's optimistic view but needed Amy's dose of reality. Both were invaluable to me."

Rori also understands the importance of having a network, particularly because she experienced what it's like *not* to have one—at the time of her oophorectomy she didn't know anyone her age who had had the same surgery for preventative reasons. "I only knew what to expect based on what the doctor had told me and what I had read online," Rori explains. "I remember being wheeled into the operating room, and I literally broke down and started crying so hard I couldn't breathe. I was terrified, and I think if I had had someone to talk to who had been through the surgery it would have allayed some of those fears. I'm just happy that I can now help Suzanne and Amy as they contemplate an oophorectomy, because I didn't have anyone."

And as the last of the five women to have a mastectomy, Suzanne says each of them helped her in different ways. "Thanks to Lisa, Mayde, Amy, and Rori, I was as prepared as someone can be for something they haven't gone through before," she says. "I knew what kind of post-mastectomy exercises I should do, what pain meds to ask for, what it is like losing sensation in your breasts, and how to deal with having to leave my daughter for the week of my surgery. By the time I consulted with my doctor the day of my mastectomy, I had no further questions. I had been over all of it with the girls."

mastectomy: what to expect during surgery

Before your surgery, your doctor will go over the exact details of the operation, which depends greatly on which particular procedure you chose, the facility where you'll be having it, and your physician's technique. Here's a general overview of what you might experience the day of the surgery:

A few hours beforehand, nurses will bring you into a pre-op holding area where you'll change into a hospital gown, possibly receive an intravenous (IV) tube, and get prepped for surgery. If you're feeling overly anxious, you can ask for a sedative. About thirty minutes before the actual operation, your breast surgeon will go over the plan with you once again. If you're having immediate reconstruction, your plastic surgeon will also come in to talk about the surgery and draw incision lines on your breasts with a marker. Your anesthesiologist will meet with you briefly, too, to discuss your medical history and figure out which anesthesia will be best for you.

Then you'll be taken into the operating room—which is typically cold—for the actual surgery. If you haven't received an IV tube yet, the anesthesiologist will insert one. Mastectomy is performed under general anesthesia, which is started through the IV tube and/or a face mask so that you're not conscious during the surgery. Once you're out, a tube is inserted down your throat to help facilitate breathing and maintain your anesthesia. In some cases, another tube called a catheter is put in your bladder to drain urine during the surgery. If you're having a flap surgery that removes tissue from your abdomen, a nurse might clip part of your pubic hair to keep the surgical site sterile.

A mastectomy that doesn't include breast reconstruction usually takes one to two hours per side. If you're having immediate breast reconstruction, the entire surgery can take between three and five hours per side (flap surgeries are usually twice as long as implant surgeries). Afterward, you're brought to the recovery room where nurses will watch your vital signs and check for any complications. You'll be hooked up to several different machines, such as ones that monitor your heart rate and blood pressure—and you'll hear a lot of beeping. You might feel lubricant on your eyes, which is sometimes applied to them so they don't become dry during the operation. Then you're taken up to your hospital room where you'll spend at least a night or two if you're having no reconstruction or implants, and three to five days if you've had a flap surgery.

mastectomy: the aftermath

HOW YOU WILL LOOK

After your surgery, you will be taken to a recovery room. If you had immediate reconstruction, your breasts will now be the size you'll wind up with (give or take a little swelling). Even with expanders, you won't be flat—you'll wake up with at least a small mound. Keep in mind that the appearance of your breasts will change over time. It can take months until they've achieved their final look. (See Chapter 11 to learn how to work with your doctor to determine what size and shape you want your breasts to be.) Here's what else you should expect to see right after the mastectomy:

Drains

After surgery, you have to drain excess fluid that comes out of the incision site—including blood and a clear fluid called serum—as quickly as possible. For that reason, there will be plastic tubes that go from near the wounds into little collapsible containers. The patient (or a trusted friend or family member) has to empty the containers as many as six times a day for up to two weeks or until there is less than an ounce of fluid draining each day. Typically, there will be one or two tubes in each breast and, if you choose flap reconstruction, one or two coming out of the flap area. If the tubes are still in when you return home, your nurse or doctor can help teach you how to take care of them and how to record the output.

For many women, the drains are the worst aspect of their surgery. "I hated the drains," says Amy. "If I moved, they'd tug at my skin, which was very painful. They were uncomfortable to sleep with, and it was gross seeing blood and fluids drain out of me day after day. I was so sick of the drains and it made such a difference once they were removed."

Bandages

After a mastectomy, your chest will have a bandage, tape, and gauze over the incision, and you'll possibly be wearing a special cotton surgical bra that holds your breasts tight. Often such compression makes patients feel more comfortable. If you've had a flap surgery, there may be very little in the way of dressings over the flap to allow for easy periodic inspection from your medical caretakers.

Stitches and Bruising

In most cases, the mastectomy incision is closed with dissolvable stitches. Such stitches, which might feel like little bumps under your skin, will typically disappear within a few weeks (though in Suzanne's case, it took a lot longer). If your doctor uses surgical staples instead, he'll remove them at the first office visit after your operation. Expect at least some bruising, which will vary greatly with each woman. Amy, for instance, says her breasts turned black and blue, then purple, then yellow. Bruising will fade gradually and disappear within a few weeks.

Scars

Mastectomies leave scars, but the size and location of them varies greatly on your surgeon, your breast size, and what kind of reconstruction you have, if any. Some surgeries leave small, light scars hidden in the breast folds, while others leave larger, more conspicuous ones that can appear red, dark pink, or purple. If you have a flap surgery, you'll have scars wherever the doctors removed the tissue. Scars will fade over time, and certain therapies can help them appear lighter and smoother. For instance, some doctors recommend massaging scars with an ointment or gel like Mederma or Scarguard MD starting about four weeks after surgery. Talk with your surgeon about which treatments she suggests.

Other Symptoms

Crusting along the incision lines or collections of blood under the skin are normal after surgery. Again, notify your doctor, who can determine if and how these effects need to be treated.

HOW YOU WILL FEEL

Of course, physical side effects of the surgery vary greatly with each patient. Here are some you *might* experience:

Anesthesia Effects

Anesthesia essentially shuts the whole body down—not just the mind—so when you "wake up" you might feel funny. Most people are groggy and disoriented after they first regain consciousness. If a tube was used to administer the anesthesia or assist with breathing, your throat might be sore. Sometimes patients feel nauseous or they actually vomit when they wake up. If that's the case, notify your nurse, who can give you anti-nausea medication. You might also have the chills as your body temperature readjusts or, as was true in Lisa's case, brief trouble urinating. Last, the anesthesia as well as pain meds can lead to constipation, so you might want to ask your doctor for stool softeners or mild laxatives if you didn't bring any with you to the hospital.

Exhaustion

A mastectomy is a major surgery, so it's no surprise that one of the most common complaints post-op is a complete lack of energy. Your body is healing and it needs time to recuperate. Experts say it can take a month or two until you start feeling less tired.

Soreness and Pain

Lisa says that after her surgery, it felt like there was an elephant sitting on top of her and that there were two hard rocks in place of where her breasts were. Implant patients in particular may feel tightness in their chests, and because the muscle is being lifted and stretched, they might feel spasms as well. If this occurs, your doctor can give you a muscle relaxant. Patients also might feel soreness and pressure on their chest and, if applicable, the area where the flap tissue was taken from. Some women don't complain of too much discomfort, thanks to a steady flow of pain medication. For instance, Amy says she was hooked up to a device that administered doses of anesthesia directly to her surgical incisions. Oftentimes patients are also given meds through their IV tubes—the women in this book, for instance, swear by a nonsteroidal anti-inflammatory drug called ketorolac (brand name Toradol). Some of them also took oxycodone (brand name Percocet) as well as Extra Strength Tylenol to ease the pain.

Phantom Feelings

As nerves regenerate, a woman might experience a tingling, itching, throbbing, or a sensation similar to pins and needles where the breast tissue used to be. This can occur whether or not the nipple is preserved, much like a person whose arm is amputated might still feel the missing limb. Ask your doctor for ways to lessen these symptoms. Most of this effect fades slowly over nine to twelve months.

Numbness

Right after a mastectomy, most women experience numbness in their breasts. However, about 60 percent of women will regain some sensation over time, estimates Andrew Salzberg, M.D., chief of plastic surgery at Westchester Medical Center in New York. "It runs the gamut, and we can't make predictions—some patients wind up with total numbness, while others have full feeling," he says. Keep in mind that nerves grow very slowly, so it can take years to get considerable feeling back.

RESUMING ACTIVITIES

Ask your doctor about when you can go back to your daily routine. On average, most experts say patients should not lift their arms above 90 degrees until the drains are out. After that, you can gradually add back activities week by week, per your physician's approval. For instance, by the second or third week you will be able to drive; by a month to six weeks you can exercise. Some doctors want their patients to refrain from showering until they no longer need drains. Instead they recommend sponge baths for a week or so. Most important, take it easy and rest as much as you can.

Post-Op Exercises

There are certain exercises you can do to help your mobility and speed recovery. Ask your nurse or the hospital's physical therapist to provide you with a routine that you should follow after your drains are removed.

POST-OP SURVEILLANCE

There are no national guidelines regarding surveillance after a prophylactic mastectomy. However, doctors will typically want to see their patients within a few weeks after the surgery, a few months down the road, and yearly thereafter. Ask your physician to teach you how to do a monthly breast self-exam now that you have a new breast "architecture," suggests Julie Margenthaler, M.D., a surgical oncologist at the Siteman Cancer Center at Washington University School of Medicine in St. Louis. "I teach my patients what to look for, like lumps along the implant, nodules in the skin, and anything that feels abnormal in the chest wall," she says. You should also have a yearly exam by your physician. As for screening, experts don't recommend doing yearly mammograms because there's almost no breast tissue left behind after a prophylactic mastectomy. However, if you have silicone implants, the FDA recommends having an MRI three years after implantation and then every two years after that to make sure the implant hasn't ruptured.

oophorectomy: before the surgery (for brca carriers)

HOW TO FIND A DOCTOR

While any gynecologic surgeon can perform an oophorectomy, many experts recommend that high-risk women see a gynecologic oncologist—a doctor specifically trained in finding cancer. The Society of Gynecologic

Oncologists can help you find such experts in your area by state or by name (www.sgo.org).

However, as mentioned earlier in this chapter, it's important to trust your instincts when choosing a doctor. For instance, Rori said that when it came time to book her oophorectomy, she interviewed several gynecologic oncologists but ultimately decided to go with her regular gynecologist instead. "I had a fifteen-year history with my gynecologist—he delivered two of my children, and I felt safe with him," she says. "I wasn't just another patient to him, and I really didn't want to go with someone I didn't know. I also knew that if, God forbid, he found anything suspicious on my ovaries, he'd have an oncologist on standby. In the end, I decided to trust my gut, and I'm glad that I did."

If you do choose to go with a gynecologist, check to make sure he or she is a member of the American College of Obstetricians and Gynecologists (www.acog.org). Their ob/gyn fellows are all board-certified. (Note: Gynecologic oncologists can be members of ACOG as well.)

QUESTIONS FOR A GYNECOLOGIST/ GYNECOLOGIC ONCOLOGIST

Along with the general questions mentioned earlier in this chapter, you might want to ask the following:

- Have you performed prophylactic oophorectomies on high-risk women?
- What are the benefits of removing my uterus along with my ovaries and tubes?
- Will you call in a gynecologic oncologist if cancer is discovered during the surgery? (If your doctor isn't one already.)
- When should I consider exploring my hormone replacement options?

- Will you perform a peritoneal wash (the pelvic cavity is bathed in a saline solution, and the fluid is then removed and examined for cancer cells)?
- Do you check the tissue you remove extra-carefully when a patient has a BRCA mutation?

WHAT TO BRING TO THE HOSPITAL

The pre-op checklists for an oophorectomy are pretty much the same as those for a mastectomy. You should also bring cotton underwear and large sanitary pads, as you might experience some vaginal bleeding and discharge after an oophorectomy. You'll also want to wear loose pants, especially if you're having a laparotomy (as described below).

oophorectomy: what to expect during surgery

If you're having your ovaries and fallopian tubes removed, much of the pre-op is similar to that for a mastectomy. Your nurse will insert an IV tube and catheter, and she'll possibly clip your pubic area.

The ins and outs of the actual surgery (called a bilateral salpingo-oophorectomy) depends on whether or not you're having a laparoscopy or a laparotomy, says Angeles Alvarez Secord, M.D., a gynecologic oncologist at Duke University Medical Center in North Carolina. Here's a breakdown of the difference between these two procedures:

Laparoscopy: In this procedure, typically done under regional or general anesthesia, the surgeon makes an incision in the belly button, through which she inserts a small camera called a laparoscope. This device allows her to see the ovaries and surrounding organs up close. She then makes a few tiny incisions around the pubic area and/or lower abdomen. The surgeon inserts tools into these incisions to surgically remove the ovaries and tubes, which are typically delivered back through the small incisions or through the vagina if a hysterectomy is being performed as well. The cuts are closed with dissolvable stitches, and the entire surgery takes between one and three hours. Many times, a laparoscopy is done as an outpatient procedure and the patient goes home the same day. If the uterus is being removed as well, most women will spend one night in the hospital.

Laparotomy: This procedure is the traditional way an oophorectomy is performed. While the minimally invasive laparoscopy might seem the preferred method, whether or not it's right for you depends on your surgeon's expertise as well as your medical history. For instance, if you have a lot of scar tissue from previous surgeries such as C-sections, a laparoscopic surgery might not be possible. In a laparotomy, typically performed under general anesthesia, the doctor makes up to a six-inch incision either horizontally across the bikini line or vertically between the belly button and pubic bone. The stomach muscles are pulled apart and the ovaries and fallopian tubes are surgically removed. The doctor will stitch up the wound, and you'll stay in the hospital for three to five days.

oophorectomy: the aftermath

HOW YOU WILL LOOK

Stitches

Most laparoscopic oophorectomies are performed with adhesive or dissolvable stitches, which disappear within a few weeks. With a laparotomy, doctors will use either absorbable stitches or staples, or metal staples that they then remove two to seven days after surgery.

Bandages
After a laparoscopy, sterile bandages cover the incision sites. Because a laparotomy requires a much larger incision, you might have gauze, tape, and other dressings, too. Typically bandages are removed within a few days after surgery.

Scars
Scars are basically as long as the incisions. So, if you've had a laparoscopic surgery, you will have about three to four little scars across your abdomen and pelvic area. If you've had a traditional laparotomy, you'll have a scar across your bikini line or from your belly button to your pubic bone.

Bruising
While women might experience bruising after an oophorectomy, it's typically minimal and disappears within one to two weeks.

HOW YOU WILL FEEL

Pain
Each patient's threshold for pain varies greatly. Some women experience very little discomfort, while others are laid up for weeks. Ask your doctor for a prescription painkiller if you need relief.

Bloating
After an oophorectomy, many women experience bloating for a few weeks. This can be due to swelling or to the fact that during a laparoscopic surgery, the abdomen is filled with gas to allow the surgeon to see and operate. Also, anesthesia and pain medication can lead to constipation, which may also cause bloating. If you experience

bloating, drink plenty of fluids and talk to your doctor about possible remedies.

Exhaustion

As with a mastectomy, recovering from a major surgery can be energy-zapping. Recovery time is a lot quicker for laparoscopic surgeries, but either way, you might feel a little tired and sore for a few weeks.

Effects from Anesthesia

Same as with a prophylactic mastectomy (see page 135).

Menopausal Symptoms

The most dramatic physical effect of an oophorectomy is that your body stops producing estrogen and progesterone. Without those hormones, a woman might start experiencing menopausal symptoms such as hot flashes, vaginal dryness, and loss of libido immediately after surgery (though some women never have any side effects at all). Talk to your doctor about options to manage these symptoms, such as estrogen replacement therapy, antidepressants, and herbal remedies.

RESUMING ACTIVITIES

After a Laparoscopy

You can shower within twenty-four hours and drive when you're off narcotics and can react effectively to emergency situations behind the wheel. If you've had a hysterectomy as well, you should avoid sex, inserting anything in your vagina, swimming, or taking baths until you get your doctor's approval at the four-to-six-week checkup.

After a Laparotomy

You shouldn't lift anything that weighs more than ten pounds for six weeks. Typically you should avoid sex or putting anything in your vagina during that time. You might not be able to drive for up to four weeks. Also, though you can shower after twenty-four hours, you should avoid baths and swimming for two to four weeks (up to six weeks if you've had a hysterectomy, too).

Post-Op Surveillance

The jury is still out as to what kind of surveillance a woman with an elevated risk for ovarian cancer should do after she's had an oophorectomy. However, because cancer can still form in the peritoneal lining or, if the patient hasn't had a hysterectomy, the uterus, many experts recommend that high-risk women still get yearly pelvic exams and CA-125 blood tests. Rori says that after her surgery, her doctor also gave her some advice. "He said I should pay attention to my body, and if I felt tired or any pain or bloating, I should see him."

psychological issues after prophylactic surgeries

SECOND GUESSING

Once Suzanne opted to have a mastectomy, she never once doubted her decision. That is, until the morning of her actual operation. "My doctors showed up late, so I was waiting outside the operating room by myself for more than two hours. I was lying there in my paper gown and just started freaking out. I was thinking, 'What am I doing? This is insane. I'm not cutting my breasts off. I'm out of here!' I actually got up and was trying to figure out how to unhook the IV, when it suddenly felt like a hand forced me down on the gurney. I swear, it's crazy, but I think it was my mother pushing me, saying, 'Lie back and don't move. You know what can happen if you don't do this.'"

No one ever said surgery was a breeze, particularly when it comes to a prophylactic procedure. While cancer patients often feel like they have no choice but to have certain operations, there can always be a window of doubt for a previvor. Rori, for instance, says that for a long time after her mastectomy she occasionally wondered if she made the right decision having the surgery. "When I had my ovaries removed, I didn't have a doubt in my mind," she says. "Ovarian cancer is a silent killer, and after seeing what it did to my mother and sister, I knew having the surgery was something I had to do. I have never second-guessed that decision for a second. But I felt differently about my breasts. I was so attached to them, and these new ones didn't feel like they were a part of me. Up until recently, I had a weird stiffness at times and little feeling. Now I feel comfortable with my breasts and I have more sensation, but at first I really questioned if I should have done surveillance instead."

However, despite some hesitations immediately before and after the surgery, in the long run most women do not regret having prophylactic mastectomies. A study in the *Journal of the American Medical Association* found that nearly three-quarters of patients who had the procedure were satisfied with it. And a separate study by the American Society of Plastic Surgeons reported that 100 percent of women who had bilateral prophylactic mastectomies were satisfied with their breast reconstruction and all would have the surgery again.

For instance, despite her fears right before surgery, afterward Suzanne didn't second-guess herself for a second. Lisa had a somewhat similar experience. "Even as they were wheeling me into surgery, I was worried whether I was doing the right thing, especially since I didn't have a BRCA gene mutation," she says. "Then that first week I was so achy and uncomfortable, I kept thinking to myself, 'I hope I didn't make the wrong decision.' But as soon as I started to feel better, I knew I hadn't."

Among the five women, Amy's situation is unique. She says while she doesn't regret her mastectomy, her perspective has changed because she's gotten divorced since her operation. "I'm happy that the surgery is over with, but I don't know if I would have done it had I known I was going to be single again," she says. "If I had a spouse, I'd be content, and I wouldn't think twice about what I did. But it's different for me now. I think about how men will react to the new me when I start dating. Will they be scared by the word 'mastectomy'?"

SAYING GOOD-BYE

Regardless of the relationship a woman has with her breasts, removing them can be a very traumatic experience. Even if a woman wasn't that emotionally attached to her breasts to begin with, she may grieve their loss both before and after her operation.

Mayde can relate. She said that the month before her surgery, she'd cry in bed at night, mourning the impending loss of her breasts. "I was worried, thinking, 'Will they lose their sensation? Will I look fake? Will I feel whole again? Will I feel normal?'" she recalls. "I also had my husband take a picture of my chest so I could compare my final results to what I looked like before the surgery."

Rori also had a difficult time right before her mastectomy, and she'd touch her breasts in the shower, trying to memorize how they felt. She had a similar sense of grief before her oophorectomy. "I remember having my last period, thinking on the one hand, 'Hooray, thank God this is the last time I'm going to have to deal with all those horrible symptoms.' But at the same time, I felt sad. To me, getting my period meant my body was working. It would be weird that, at thirty-eight years old, I would never menstruate again. So, knowing this was going to be my last period, I almost tried to embrace it and remember the feeling of cramping and bloating. It might sound weird, but I was so worried I'd feel empty inside afterward."

Of course, not every woman having a prophylactic surgery feels a sense of loss.

Suzanne says she was actually excited. "I didn't cry or get upset during the weeks before my surgery because I knew my breasts would probably look better than ever, and I was so happy to be rid of my risk," she says. "I wanted to run into that operation room." Amy adds that she felt more empowered by her impending surgery than saddened. "I knew I had made the right choice, and I was confident and strong," she says. "The day of the operation, I felt like Superwoman. I woke up and thought, 'Let's just get this over with already.'"

As for Lisa, she says she didn't grieve over her breasts because she didn't feel like she was losing them. "I was having a skin-sparing surgery, so to me I was just removing cells and getting rid of my risk," Lisa says. "Everything else remained intact. I viewed it as though my breasts were faulty, and I was getting them fixed. I didn't think I was giving up anything. I was gaining peace of mind. I was surprised, however, that within three weeks after the surgery, life was back to normal, business as usual. I had been planning and anticipating my mastectomy for months, and I was amazed how quickly it was over with."

A HUGE VOID

When a woman opts to have a prophylactic surgery, it's often because she has witnessed a loved one—particularly her mother—battle the disease she's hoping to prevent. And previvors often say that one of the most difficult aspects of going through such a major preventative measure is when their moms aren't by their side.

Lisa says she broke down right before her surgery. "I was waiting on the gurney outside the operating room, and I started sobbing," she recalls. "All I could think about was my mother. I was going in for the biggest surgery of my life, and I needed her to hold my hand and help me get through this. I needed to hear her say that I was doing the right thing."

Suzanne felt the same way, and she sensed that her mother, as well as her father, was watching over her the entire time she was combating her risk. "I always felt my parents were present through this whole ordeal, and that they sent people to help me because they couldn't," she says. "First they sent me Mayde, who drove thirty minutes both ways so her daughter could take a one-hour tap class in my studio. I'm normally in such a rush at the end of class and have no time to talk, but for some reason I connected with Mayde and we wound up discussing BRCA testing. Then, when my insurance company didn't want to cover my surgery, Dr. Salzberg and his office manager, Beth, got on the phone to fight for me even though I barely knew them. These people are angels on Earth, and I know my parents put them in my path."

Even for women whose mothers survived cancer, it can be difficult reliving the experience. "My mother's mastectomy was horrific—she almost died and was left flat, scarred, and in chronic pain," explains Mayde. "So when I told my mother I was electively having a mastectomy, she said, 'Why would you want to put yourself through this? Do you think it's going to be easy, because it's not.' Then, as I was planning my trip to New York for my surgery, she didn't even volunteer to come with me. I think psychologically she couldn't handle going through a mastectomy again. But a few days before my operation, I was so nervous that my husband called my mother and told her that I would need her at the hospital. My mother wound up coming, and what struck me most was her reaction following my surgery. A few hours after the operation, I was conscious, sitting up in bed and talking on my cell phone, not drugged up and writhing in pain like she was when she had her mastectomy. I had no bruising, and my breasts looked great. She turned to my surgeon and said, 'Is this for real? She looks amazing.' My mom had been so afraid that I'd suffer the way she did, and she was both shocked and relieved when she realized I was fine."

RELYING ON OTHERS

Just as it helps to build a network before your surgery, it can also make a huge difference having that same support system in place while you're recovering. "When you return home, you feel so helpless," says Lisa. "You can't carry anything or lift your arms, and you're mostly stuck home trying to get better. I remember I once called one of my friends, crying, because I couldn't put my bra on. She came right over to help me. Neighbors and girlfriends took me food shopping, brought over dinner for my family, and drove my kids to and from school and their extracurricular activities. Amy would often come over just to keep me company or take me for a walk around the block. And my husband helped by cleaning my drains, brushing my hair, assisting me in and out of the bathtub, and holding down the fort at home. I'm not one to ask for help, but I quickly realized I had no choice. I was beyond exhausted and needed time to heal."

Rori says that friends and family also helped her with everything from laundry and cooking dinner to cleaning up the house, but very few people could help her emotionally. At that point, Rori had met Mayde through FORCE, and says that she was her lifeline. "After my mastectomy, Mayde was the only person I could talk to about what positions to sleep in, how to prop up my arms, and how long I'd have bruising and swelling," Rori says.

Suzanne adds that while Lisa, Mayde, Amy, and Rori all guided her before her surgery, she didn't feel like she needed as much help after the fact. "After my mastectomy, I made sure my husband called all the girls, letting them know I was okay," she says. "And while they talked me through any issues I may have had over the next few weeks, I really felt great for the most part. At that point, I mostly wanted the four of them to celebrate with me. No one else could fully understand what I had been through and what it meant to me that my surgery was now behind me."

ONE PREVIVOR'S ACCOUNT

While every woman's experience having a prophylactic surgery is unique, Rori dealt with many of the same issues addressed in this chapter and wrote about them in a journal. Here's what she was actually thinking and feeling the first week after her mastectomy:

June 14, 2006: I just woke up from my surgery and barely remember much, except for feeling a huge sense of relief and calmness. I'm thinking back to where I just came from, where I was, and what I was doing. I'm not really in pain, but I'm tired. It's all a blur.

June 15, 2006: I feel sick and nauseous, but I'm so happy. It's done! It's over! I can't believe I really did this. My fear is gone, but I'm throwing up! I'm not feeling too good today.

June 16, 2006: Yesterday, they finally gave me an anti-nausea shot, so today I feel like a new person. I can actually eat, sit up, and walk around the entire floor. And most important, I can have my hair washed. Yay! I had the most wonderful nurse today. I wish I could remember her name. I have her beautiful smile pictured in my memory. She has no idea how much she helped me.

June 17, 2006: I'm home. Well, not actually home, but in New York City to stay for the next week and let this entire process sink in. Those dreaded drains are the worst part. I brought my husband's button downs so I would have big, baggy, comfy shirts. Last night, we went out for Thai food at our favorite restaurant and walked around. I then went back to our room, took a pain pill, and went to sleep.

June 18, 2006: The morning and the early nights are most difficult. I feel uncomfortable, stiff, and just plain yucky. I use a lot of pillows in bed and always take my pain medication every few hours because I don't want to be in pain. My husband has been an amazing help to me. Not only was Terry by my side through these decisions, my consultations, and my surgeries, but he has also been draining my drains each day, helping me shower and get dressed, washing and drying my hair. He even ran to a Gap and brought me some more baggy shirts. We've been out everywhere. And I mean everywhere: we went out to eat, walked around Central Park, saw a Broadway show and the Statue of Liberty. Nothing has stopped me. I'm exhausted at the end of the day, but we come back to our room, rest, and then venture out again at night for dinner.

June 20, 2006: My meltdown day. I woke up this morning and was not in a good mood. I was exhausted, probably from doing too much. I told my husband I wanted to stay in all day, but that he should go out and enjoy his day. I wanted to be alone. My mind started to wander. Did I make a mistake? Should I have just continued with surveillance? What did I do!? I was in the hotel room alone and I finally decided to look at my new breasts. I went into the bathroom, and when I took off my bra for the first time, I couldn't breathe. I was amazed at how good my breasts already looked and felt, even though I'm still sore and there are red marks on one of them.

I also thought about my mom today. After five years of surgeries and chemo, my mother decided to stop treatment and go out her way with her dignity. We all knew that that year was to be our last everything with our mother. The last Hanukkah, the last birthdays and Thanksgiving. We took our last family photo. Toward the end of her life, my mother deteriorated quite rapidly. She became a shell of her existence. She knew that when her hospice came and her deathbed was delivered, it was the end. I'll never forget the day we put my mother in that bed, she just wanted to be gone already. She hated the slow, painful process of dying. On April 19, 1997, at 9:27 p.m., my mother took her last breath with a tear streaming down her face. I've never been the same since, and I never will be.

Rori says that when she returned home from her surgery, she didn't have time to write in her journal. But in retrospect, she says, "Once I was home and starting to recover, I was able to sit back and reflect on my surgeries and my journey. I thought about all those biopsies, tests, and consultations I went through. I thought about what my mother had endured and what I had done to make sure that I wouldn't suffer the same fate. I had done everything I could to lower my risk, and couldn't believe that I no longer had the fear I had always lived with. I felt such a sense of peace, and was so relieved it was finally over."

love, sex, and babies

"My husband, Terry, was never one of those fake-boob men," says Rori. "He always loved the look and feel of natural breasts, and I happened to be very well-endowed. However, when I told him I was considering a mastectomy, he backed me one hundred percent. Terry was affectionate and supportive, and promised to take care of the house, the kids, anything I needed to get through this whole ordeal. Right after my surgery, he seemed to like my new breasts, but our intimacy changed. I had always been less inhibited, and it upset Terry that I didn't get the same pleasure from my breasts anymore. He still touched them when we made love, but it was weird for me, because I had light tingling in some areas and in others I couldn't feel a thing. Over time, my breasts started feeling more a part of me and our sex life eventually returned to normal, but we certainly went through a rough patch at first."

When a woman considers ways to fight her risk of cancer, her actions will often affect current or future relationships. And the reverse is true, too—a woman's love life, sex life, and whether or not she's had children can greatly influence her decision in the first place. "In a surprising percentage of cases, when a patient is stuck on what course of action to take, it's because she's worried her current or future partner will react negatively to certain choices," says Paul Jacobsen, Ph.D., chair of the department of health outcomes and behavior at Moffitt Cancer Center in Tampa. However, having a supportive other half can make this experience run a lot smoother. "Couples who are committed and have good means of communication take this in stride as they would other stressful situations," Dr. Jacobsen explains.

Whether you're single, dating, in a serious relationship, or married, the degree to which the issues in this book might impact your love life runs the gamut. The good news is that the vast majority of couples will make it through. But that doesn't mean it might not be difficult at times.

the role of a relationship

STRENGTHENING A SOLID FOUNDATION

As with any life crisis, dealing with breast cancer risk can make a relationship stronger. "When a woman in a stable relationship is considering genetic testing, increased surveillance, or ways to reduce her odds of getting breast cancer, that experience can bring her and her partner closer together," says Mary Jane Massie, M.D., a psychiatrist who counsels high-risk women at Memorial Sloan-Kettering Cancer Center in New York City. "If a patient's partner is coming to her doctor appointments and talking through the issues with her, it proves to the woman that her significant other really does love her and support her decisions."

Suzanne agrees. "Going through BRCA testing and my mastectomy solidified the bond between my husband, Pascal, and me just like my infertility treatments, my father's death, and other traumatic experiences have done," she says. "Each time, we've strengthened our marriage and confirmed that we will stick by each other in sickness and in health. For example, when my BRCA results were in, my husband insisted on coming with me to my counselor's office, and he held my hand while I received the news. Then he joined me on interviews with doctors and, for the two months before my mastectomy, he took care of shopping, cleaning, and caring for our daughter so I could focus on getting ready for the surgery. Of course, he came to New York for my operation and, afterward, he did everything from emptying my drains and bathing me to cooking dinner for our family. Knowing he was there for me made it so much easier to get through this nightmare."

Lisa says that her husband, Bob, was also extremely helpful and that when it came to her risk they were truly "in this together." "My husband had been living with my fear of breast cancer since we started dating," Lisa explains. "He experienced the panic that came with every mammogram, every lump, and every biopsy. He was there when my mother passed away and he was devastated by her loss. So when Bob realized a prophylactic mastectomy would alleviate all of our concerns, he was completely on board. And because I didn't have my mother by my side, I needed that support from Bob even more."

Lisa notes that removing the fear has also strengthened her marriage. "Breast cancer was such a big part of our relationship, but not anymore," she says. "We both have so much less anxiety, and we no longer have to focus on this terrible disease. The decision to have a mastectomy was as much for Bob and my three children as it was for me."

A DIFFICULT ROAD

While getting through any stressful situation can make a marriage or serious relationship stronger, it can also tear a couple apart. "Couples who have problems to begin with are more likely to have difficulty dealing with high-risk issues," explains Dr. Jacobsen. "The stress acts as a kind of amplifier. It can make whatever is good in the relationship better, but it can also make whatever is bad in the relationship worse."

Amy can relate. When she tested positive for a BRCA mutation and later had a prophylactic mastectomy, she was married and her husband at the time was supportive and attentive to her needs. However, a year and a half after her surgery they separated, and Amy questions if stress played a part in that. "Having the BRCA mutation, doing research on my options, flying to New York for my surgery—maybe my ex-husband got overwhelmed with everything I was going through," she says. "I don't regret what I did, and I don't want to blame my BRCA mutation for the failure of my marriage. There were certainly other factors involved. But right after that whole ordeal is when things started falling apart. I know I can't turn back the clock, but I wonder what would have happened if I never got tested."

While Amy's problems with her husband manifested *after* her surgery, it can be equally as distressing if a woman's partner is not on the same page with her while she's in the throws of first deciding how to tackle her risk. A study in the *American Journal of Medical Genetics*, for instance, found that women who tested positive for a genetic mutation were considerably more likely to experience distress if their partners were anxious and nonsupportive. And though she was BRCA-negative, Mayde agrees that planning for her mastectomy put stress on her marriage—especially when her husband initially doubted her decision (in part because she *didn't* have the genetic mutation). Mayde recalls, "At first, Jonathan was trying to persuade me not to have the surgery by having me talk to his colleagues who also thought a mastectomy was a crazy idea. I was pissed off. This was a choice *I* had made! And while I understand that Jonathan is a radiologist and coming at this from a medical perspective, I just wanted him to be a supportive husband. It became an ongoing debate. Once we were meeting with a breast surgeon, and I noticed Jonathan was trying to egg the doctor on and twist his answers so that it would seem like the doctor didn't approve of my having the surgery. That almost caused an all-out war. I was thinking, 'Don't you dare try to impose your views. I'm here for an unbiased opinion.' Later, when I went for counseling to help deal with all of the issues I was going through, the biggest topic the therapist and I discussed was how to handle Jonathan. He couldn't relinquish control and just be there for me. It put such a strain on us at the time."

Experts say there are ways to ward off any negative effects that dealing with a high risk for cancer can have on a relationship. One of the biggest tips: Get your significant other involved from the get-go, says Dr. Jacobsen. "When a partner doesn't accompany a woman on the day she gets the results from a BRCA test, for instance, it may be a sign of poor communication," he says. While making major decisions about risk, it's important to educate your loved one and discuss *both* of your concerns. Ask him to join you at doctor appointments and let him ask questions, too. By talking about these issues *before* you make any decisions, you can figure out what all the physical, emotional, and financial repercussions might be with options such as surgery. Then you can work through any potential problems prior to making major life changes. And you might also consider seeking professional help—in Mayde's case, talking with a therapist helped her work through her problems with her husband. "Jonathan was really trying to steer my medical course, and my therapist helped me learn how to remind him that I was in charge of my own health and body," she says.

SINGLE AND DATING

While being in a relationship can greatly affect how a woman handles her risk, *not* being in one can have a much more dramatic impact. Most experts agree that single women are the hardest hit when dealing with a high risk for breast cancer because this demographic has a whole slew of unique issues to face. Some feel rushed to fall in love, get married, and have babies so they can then have their breasts and/ or ovaries removed. To them, a clock is constantly ticking.

"All women dealing with risk and having prophylactic surgeries have to ask themselves if they'll be able to live with their decisions, but for single women, there are different questions, fears, and uncertainties on the table," says Lindsay Avner, founder of Bright Pink, a nonprofit organization for young women who are high risk for breast and/or ovarian cancer. "They also have to ask themselves if someone else who hasn't even met them yet will be able to live with this, too." In other words, women in healthy relationships already have partners to provide unconditional love. The single girl has to wonder if having a high risk for cancer or, more specifically, having a genetic mutation that can be passed on to children will scare off potential life partners. Will her having multiple biopsies, taking chemopreventive drugs, or undergoing a mastectomy or oophorectomy be too much for someone else to handle? Will these issues prevent her from living "happily ever after"?

Though Amy was married when she had her surgery, now she's single and has a new perspective on what she went through and how it might affect her future. "I had a very telling experience on the first date I had after I was separated," she says. "Mayde set me up with a guy she knows. He knew about her surgery, but not about mine. Anyway, during the date we were making small talk, discussing how we both knew Mayde. Referring to her mastectomy, he said, 'Don't you think it's a little extreme what Mayde did?' I told him I had the same surgery, and he just got very quiet. It was then that I realized that dating was going to be a big challenge. Some men probably won't be too fazed by what I did, while others will think I'm crazy. It's certainly not something I'm going to bring up right away."

In fact, deciding *when* to tell a new boyfriend or significant other is a major concern for many single girls. Some women think that unloading such a big issue may scare someone off. Others are worried that doing so will pressure the relationship to advance to the next level. Lindsay Avner says it's a very individual decision. "You might feel like you want to blurt this out right away, so that if a guy wants to run, he can; but that's really not necessary," she says. "You have to wait until the time is right and you feel ready to share this news with him. For some women, that might be on a second date; for others it might be months into the relationship. Just remember that you are a dynamic person and this is just one part of who you are."

Another aspect of being single is that women are afraid of being called "high-risk" because they're afraid that such a label will affect their appeal to the opposite sex. Amy understands this all too well. "When I was married, I didn't think twice about testing and having my surgery," she says. "I had a husband. He was going to love me no matter what. But now that I'm single and dating, I wonder whether men will judge me (though someone who does is clearly not the right person for me). I'm glad I went through with it all, but I don't know if I would have if I had been single at the time." Adds Lisa, "I recently met a girl named Jennifer who is single, thirty-seven years old, and just tested positive for BRCA2. She plans on not telling anyone about her BRCA status except for the man she winds up marrying. In her mind, it's a private matter and no one's business but her own."

Of course, there are plenty of men who *will* love a woman regardless of what she's been through. But from the point of view of single women, they sometimes think their risk or the fact that they had a major surgery will prevent their dreams from coming true, says Elsa Reich, a genetic counselor at New York University School of Medicine. "They wonder, 'How will I ever find someone to love me?'" she explains. "The truth is, this isn't the end of the world. But it sometimes seems as if it is." On message boards and blogs, many women attest to the fact that finding love *is* possible. For instance, one woman who had a prophylactic mastectomy said she has since started dating someone who accepts her "as whole" even though her surgical results were far from perfect. Men like that *do* exist, she attests. Another woman says that after her surgery she thought she'd be single the rest of her life—that is, until she met the man she eventually married. And then Reich tells of a young woman who was diagnosed with breast cancer and planning to have bilateral mastectomies. Right before her surgery, her boyfriend whisked her away for a quick getaway to Europe. On the plane ride home, he proposed.

LET'S TALK ABOUT SEX

One way or another, dealing with a high risk for breast cancer can greatly affect a couple's intimacy. Regardless of whether you choose surveillance, chemoprevention, or a prophylactic surgery, the stress alone of deciding on a course of action can wreak havoc on your sex life. "When a woman is trying to prevent a potentially fatal disease and she becomes preoccupied with figuring out what to do, sex can slip way down to the bottom of the priority scale," explains Ralph Alterowitz, a sexuality counselor in Potomac, Maryland, and a cofounder of the Center for Intimacy After Cancer Therapy. "Many women don't even think about making love, because they're so focused on what they consider a matter of survival."

Then, after a woman makes a decision on how to combat her risk, that choice can also have a direct physiological impact on her enjoyment of sex. Premenopausal women who take tamoxifen may experience vaginal dryness as one of the side effects. And, for women who have prophylactic surgeries, there are physical barriers—after a mastectomy or an oophorectomy, a doctor might tell his patient that she *shouldn't* have sex until the follow-up appointment. And even after he's given his approval for hopping back in the sack, a woman might face other physical issues such as numbness in her breasts, discomfort or, in the case of an oophorectomy, vaginal dryness and a loss of libido.

There can be a psychological aftermath, too. As for surveillance, Suzanne attests, "When I was waiting for my results after each mammogram, sex was the very last thing on my mind." And post-mastectomy, resuming sex can actually be traumatic for some women, says Altero-witz. "After this surgery, a woman might not feel particularly sexy anymore, or she might be worried that her partner will perceive her as less feminine," he says. "Also, her significant other's reaction plays a huge part of the equation, especially if he or she doesn't want to caress or touch her reconstructed breasts for any reason."

Of course, not all women experience such physical and emotional effects, but plenty of previvors do. Rori, for one, says her breasts were always a very important part of her intimacy, but things changed after her mastectomy. "At first, I took a while getting comfortable with the 'new me' and I often wore a bra to bed for a few months," she says. "And even though I'm not self-conscious about my breasts anymore, I don't get the same pleasure from them because I'm numb in some areas."

However, Rori adds that having her ovaries removed affected her sex life much more than her mastectomy did. "After my surgery, I had to wait six weeks before I had sex," she says. "But even after I got the okay from my doctor, I had such little desire and vaginal dryness. My husband, Terry, and I tried to have sex, but it was so painful from the dryness that I started to cry. Terry was supportive and understand-ing, but all I could think was, 'How are we going to survive having a sexless marriage?' I was determined to find help. After a bit of trial and error, I came across a low-estrogen vaginal ring that helped with lubrication and was a total lifesaver. I also started natural hormone replacement therapy, which worked wonders for my libido. Within a few months, our sex life was much better. But that was a very difficult time for us."

Like Rori, Lisa says that sex has changed in some ways because her breasts are so sensitive in some areas that if her husband touches them, she jumps. Other parts of her breasts feel numb. "Bob was actually a little afraid to touch me at first, and now I have to guide him to 'touch me here, not there,'" she says. On the other hand, Lisa adds that her operation has also improved her intimacy because her husband is thrilled with the results. "Bob is a happy camper," she says. "He's always been somewhat of a 'breast man' and was more involved with choosing a cup size than with any other aspect of my surgery. Now he thinks I look fantastic and loves my slightly bigger, perkier breasts. It's like he has new toys to play with."

Keep in mind that in many cases when a woman's sex life is negatively affected by her mastectomy, it's not because her partner is unhappy with the cosmetic results. Often a woman's deflated body image and newfound fears about her sexuality are what ultimately affect the physical relationship.

SEX AND THE SINGLE GIRL

Sex with a new partner is very different from sex in a long-term relationship, primarily because the familiarity and comfort level usually aren't as high. So it makes sense that any effects surveillance or risk-reducing options might have on a woman's sex life can be magnified when she's first dating someone. Amy, for one, says that she never worried about how her breasts looked or felt after her surgery because she was married at the time. But now that she's single, she's concerned men will look at her differently. "Dating is going to be difficult no matter what, but I'll probably be even more self-conscious because I not only come with a genetic mutation, but I also have fake boobs and can't feel a thing," she says.

Lindsay Avner of Bright Pink agrees that, initially, many women ask themselves questions like: "Am I going to scare men away?" "Will I ever be attractive to anyone again?" "Will I ever feel sexy again?" Often, she says, it takes only "one experience of being with a man who is all-embracing and warm and wonderful to get past that. That definitive moment sets the stage for the woman to move forward. Her mind-set shifts from insecurity to realizing that she isn't broken or damaged. She realizes that everything is going to be okay."

TIPS ON IMPROVING INTIMACY

You can get back in the groove, but sometimes it takes a little work. Here's what you and your partner can do to help reestablish a healthy sex life:

TALK ABOUT IT

Whether you're dealing with the results of a genetic test, deciding how you want to reduce your risk of getting cancer, or actually undergoing a prophylactic surgery, communication is the key to maintaining closeness with your partner, experts say. It's important that you tell each other what you're thinking and feeling each step of the way, says Hani Miletski, Ph.D., a sex therapist in Bethesda, Maryland. Once you open up those lines of communication, you'll be better able to discuss sex and how it might be different after, say, a mastectomy. Otherwise sex becomes the "big elephant in the room no one is talking about," says Dr. Miletski.

If you're having trouble getting your partner to open up about sex, establish a bridge, experts suggest. Some couples barely communicate about anything at all, so it's important to talk about politics, sports, anything that starts a dialogue. Then you can gradually shift the conversation over to more intimate or serious topics.

GET PHYSICAL

Skin is one of the largest sex organs in the body, so spend time during the day touching, kissing, and holding hands. Doing so introduces sensuality back into the relationship without the pressure of having intercourse. And eventually that physicality can translate to the bedroom.

FIND A NEW REPERTOIRE

After a major surgery like a mastectomy, some couples have to learn how to have sex with each other again. This can be a great opportunity to rejuvenate and reshape your sexual life, and figure out what works now and what doesn't. For instance, you might want to try different positions during intercourse to find out which ones are most comfortable. Also, your partner can explore your body to figure out which areas now give you pleasure.

MAKE YOURSELF COMFORTABLE

If you're insecure about your new breasts or any scars, you can either dim the lights and stay under the covers or wear a camisole or negligee during sex until you're comfortable revealing your body to your partner. A slinky outfit might even help spice things up!

GET LUBRICATED

There are ways to overcome any vaginal dryness you might experience because of chemoprevention or an oophorectomy. Ask your doctor to suggest remedies such as the vaginal ring, which was "a total lifesaver" for Rori. Over-the-counter water-based lubricants like K-Y Jelly and Astroglide can also help.

JUST DO IT . . .

What's critical is that intimacy returns at some point, says Dr. Jacobsen. "Some couples get stuck in a rut, and the longer they don't have sex, the worse the outcome will be," he explains. "With persistent lack of intimacy, other lines of communication break down, and that can cause a vicious downward spiral." Of course, sometimes that's easier said than done, especially when certain preventative options can destroy libido. However, experts say that sometimes it's mind over matter—a woman may not think she wants sex, but if her partner initiates foreplay, she might actually get turned on. An important note: If sex is ever painful or uncomfortable in any way, you should stop and call your doctor. And in the meantime, find other ways to be intimate without having intercourse.

ASK FOR HELP

If you're having trouble getting back in the sack and you and your partner need guidance on how to talk about it, a "sexpert" can help you work through your issues. Contact the American Association of Sexuality Educators, Counselors and Therapists (AASECT) to find someone in your area who can assist you (www.aasect.org).

biological clocks and babies

When a woman has a high risk for breast cancer due to a BRCA gene mutation, it means she has a high risk for ovarian cancer as well. As previously discussed, the most effective way a previvor can reduce that risk is by having her ovaries removed. However, for many women who haven't finished or even started their family, the pressure to have that surgery is overwhelming, especially for those who haven't found a partner yet. "It's a very scary concept that you might lose your ability to have kids," says Lindsay Avner of Bright Pink. "Young women have to ask themselves questions like, 'If I don't find Mr. Right, do I want to become a parent on my own?' or 'Should I harvest my eggs or find a sperm donor and freeze my embryos?' All women have a time limit on when they can have children, but for those with a BRCA mutation, that time line is on caffeine." Of course, a woman can do surveillance, and then if she decides to have an oophorectomy, she can do so when she feels the time is right for *her*. It's a highly personal decision.

RUSHING INTO MOTHERHOOD

Some medical providers tell their patients that if they have a BRCA mutation, they need to have their ovaries removed by age thirty-five or forty. As for Rori, she already had her family and was done having children, so she could rationalize having the surgery at age thirty-eight. However, for women who haven't had children yet, this news can be devastating. Lisa's friend Jennifer, who tested positive for BRCA2, told Lisa she's "freaking out" about her risk for ovarian cancer. Jen says she wants to have an oophorectomy, but she also wants to get pregnant someday. She explained to Lisa that she feels like she's on a time clock, but she'd give up her chances to have biological kids if it meant possibly saving her life.

Of course, each woman's approach to prophylactic surgeries varies greatly based on her specific concerns and fertility needs. Some women clearly want to get childbearing over with so they can proceed with risk-reducing therapies, while many others figure they'll wait to have the surgery until they're ready on their own terms, says Lee Shulman, M.D., head of the reproductive genetics division at the Feinberg School of Medicine at Northwestern University in Chicago.

Dr. Shulman, who is also a co-director of the Ovarian Cancer Early Detection and Prevention Program at Northwestern Memorial Hospital, adds that while some women feel an internal pressure, sometimes their doctors are quick to push them into surgery. "It's true that the sooner you remove your ovaries and breasts, the sooner you'll reduce your risk of certain cancers, but it's important to remember that women are much more than just those body parts," he says. "While the surgeries will leave you with a marked reduction of cancer, you may also then have an avalanche of menopausal symptoms, infertility, and self-esteem issues." In other words, it's crucial to weigh the costs of certain surgeries. As Dr. Shulman puts it, "Life is more than cancer risk, and for some women, the effects of risk reduction might not be acceptable."

PREIMPLANTATION GENETIC DIAGNOSIS

If a woman or man carries a BRCA1 or BRCA2 genetic mutation, there's a 50/50 chance she or he will pass it on to each child. However, women contemplating having babies can go through a process called preimplantation genetic diagnosis (PGD) to increase the chances their offspring won't inherit those particular mutations (or hundreds of others linked to diseases such as cystic fibrosis, Tay-Sachs disease, and Huntington's disease). The process is complicated and costly—it requires a woman to go through in vitro fertilization, which can cost tens of thousands of dollars out-of-pocket per round, while PGD tacks on an extra few thousand to the bill.

Here's how it works: Women will have a select number of eggs removed, which are then fertilized outside the uterus in a Petri dish with a partner's (or donor's) sperm. The fertilized eggs become embryos. When those embryos are still in an early stage (usually three to five days), one cell will be removed from each and tested to see if it carries a BRCA mutation. Then the parents can decide to implant only the embryos *without* a mutation back into the mother's uterus or they can freeze them for later use. As for the affected embryos, many women choose to store and save them, says Gwendolyn Quinn, Ph.D., principal investigator of the Moffitt Fertility Preservation Group in Tampa. This process is highly accurate, though it's not entirely foolproof—false positives and false negatives are possible.

PGD is at the center of an ethically charged debate. For one, some experts argue that when a person has a genetic mutation for disorders like Tay-Sachs disease and Huntington's disease, there's a 100 percent chance he or she will have the disease from birth. However, there's no guarantee that people with BRCA mutations will develop breast cancer and, even if they do, it's typically later in life. Also, there's the argument that doctors are "playing God" and that allowing such testing can create a slippery slope. The question is: What comes next?

Another issue to consider is that DNA testing can adversely affect a woman's ability to get pregnant if the embryo is harmed in any way. PGD may reduce the odds of pregnancy because the procedure requires puncturing the embryo to retrieve the cell that will be used for genetic testing. If only IVF is performed but no testing, there is no need to puncture the embryo.

Ultimately, more education on this topic is needed. Women have a right to pursue PGD, but they often get incorrect, insufficient, or overly biased information about it. Some people, for instance, think the purpose of this technology is to create a super-race—they argue that if couples can select embryos free of genetic mutations, who's to say that we won't eventually try to design "perfect" babies with desirable traits such as beauty, intelligence, and athletic ability. However, Dr. Quinn coauthored a study published in *Fertility and Sterility* that found that although 68 percent of the respondents have never heard of PGD, 57 percent believed it was an acceptable option for high-risk women and 74 percent thought that such individuals should be given information about it. Further research has shown that while some women felt cheated because they didn't know about PGD, others didn't want the technology to exist. Those in the latter group took it personally and made comments like, "If PGD had been an option thirty years ago when my mother was starting her family, I might not be here today," says Dr. Quinn.

GIVING UP BREAST-FEEDING

Removing your ovaries obviously has a much greater impact on your future as a parent than does removing your breasts. However, a mastectomy does affect one important aspect of motherhood—women who have the operation will no longer be able to breast-feed. And experts say that adds another element to an already complex decision. "Women have to go through a thought process," says Dr. Quinn. "On the one hand, they think, 'I don't want to give up nursing,' but on the other they contemplate, 'If I'm not here, the question of even having children won't be an option at all.' They have to ask themselves, 'Do I breast-feed for a few years and slightly increase my odds of getting cancer or do I have the surgery right away?' It's like playing the stock market—these women have to figure out where to hedge their bets and what risks they're willing to take."

Many women don't question giving up the chance to breast-feed—for instance, Lisa's friend Jennifer told her that not breast-feeding in the future wasn't an issue at all when she decided to have a mastectomy. Others say they mourn the loss of the bonding experience, while some, like Rori, wouldn't even contemplate the prophylactic surgery until they were done having kids. "If I hadn't already had my children, I absolutely would have continued surveillance and waited to have a mastectomy so that I could breast-feed them," Rori says. "I felt a very strong need and desire to nurse my babies, but I know it's not for everyone. It's a very personal decision."

bottom line: it's about you

It's important to keep in mind that any intimate relationship is multifaceted. Dealing with your risk for breast cancer—regardless of your decision—likely is not going to be the one factor that holds you and your partner together or pulls you apart. However, it can play a role, and its ripple effect will be unique for each couple. In many ways, it's how the experience changes *you* that translates to any such transformation. For instance, some women feel so empowered after going through this whole ordeal that afterward they gather the strength to leave unhealthy or dead-end relationships.

Even single women can gain such a sense of confidence by what they've been through that they realize their own self-worth—with or without a man. "Yes, I'm worried about dating in the future, and I hope I can find someone who likes me for me," says Amy. "But if someone can't look past my genetics or past the fact that I had a mastectomy, I don't want them anyway. If I knew a man's father had had a heart attack and he himself had high blood pressure, would I not date him because he might develop heart disease someday? To me, that's ridiculous."

Any way this experience makes you stronger will only, in turn, make your relationship stronger. Mayde says that was the case with her and her husband. "Jonathan normally tries to make all the decisions in our family, so it was empowering for me that this time I made a choice that he respected in the end," she says. "Actually, I overheard him several times telling friends and colleagues on the phone how I found my surgical procedure and team of doctors on my own. He seemed really proud of me." Adds Suzanne, "I refused to sit around waiting to get cancer, and my husband, Pascal, was thrilled that I took control. It meant so much to me that he was confident that I was doing the right thing. We were in this together, we made decisions together, and we made it through this together."

But remember, regardless of your relationship status, this is your body, your health, and ultimately your decision. And *nobody* should convince you otherwise.

breast obsession and body image

Breasts, boobs, melons, tits, knockers, jugs, mounds, bust, gazongas, the twins, the girls, chi-chis, hooters, ta-tas, boobies, funbags, and one helluva rack. Whatever you want to call them, there's no escaping it—we are a breast-crazed society. In fact, type "breast" into Google and you'll get more than 85 million hits ("boobs" has nearly 40 million). Hooters, a popular fast-food chain, boasts more than 450 restaurants worldwide—its success is partially a result of the company's simple concept of hiring buxom waitresses and dressing them in tight tops. According to the American Society of Plastic Surgeons, breast augmentation is the most popular surgical cosmetic procedure in the United States, with 307,230 surgeries performed in 2008. And Guinness World Records added "Largest Augmented Breasts" as a new category in 2005. The bra size of the record holder: 42M.

So when a woman electively opts to have a mastectomy, it's not just a medical decision. It's a choice that can come with major emotional, psychological, and even societal ramifications. Also, a woman's own reaction depends on how she views her breasts, what kind of reconstruction she chooses, if any, and even where in the country she lives.

an evolving relationship

Part of a woman's feelings toward having a prophylactic mastectomy depends on her emotional attachment to her breasts. Breasts are unique in that, unlike other body parts, many women actually have a relationship with them. "Some people think that their breasts are what makes them special and what defines them as a woman," says Christine Laronga, M.D., medical director of the Comprehensive Breast Clinic at Moffitt Cancer Center in Tampa. "Others don't care much about them one way or another." And then there are those women with a high risk for breast cancer who view their breasts in a negative light—they feel like these body parts have somehow betrayed them.

Suzanne, for instance, says that her breasts always brought her more pain than pleasure. "My breasts have been an issue for me since I was a child," she explains. "For as long as I can remember, I figured that because my mother died of breast cancer, my breasts would kill me, too. Also, I started gymnastics classes when I was about eight, and in that sport, small boyish bodies are ideal and somewhat of a requirement. We'd hear in the gym, 'So and so just got her period. She's getting too big. Her gymnastics days are over.' And frequently girls would be put on probation and told, 'Lose five pounds or you're off the team.' So growing breasts wasn't viewed as the normal part of maturity that it is—in our world, when your breasts got bigger it meant that your teacher was going to say you gained weight. As for me, I used my breasts as a gauge—if they grew, that meant I needed to go on a diet.

"Other girls in my school were excited when they started to develop," Suzanne continues. "I remember one friend even stuffed socks in her bras. I was horrified. All I could think was, 'You're all so happy about this, but I hate it.' During the day, I'd wear super-tight tank tops to hide my breasts. At night, I'd lie in bed trying to flatten myself out with my hands. I wished my breasts would just disappear.

"Even though I loved gymnastics, I quickly realized I didn't have the kind of body to be successful in it. I decided to focus all of my efforts on dance instead. That sport, however, wasn't much better for me in terms of helping my body image. By the time I was twenty, I was dancing at resorts and living on coffee, cigarettes, and one can of tuna fish a day. I was skeletal, but I knew I'd be fired if I didn't fit into my costumes. But then I fell in love, got married, and started realizing that I couldn't live like this anymore. For one, I was more mature and realized how ridiculous it was that I was killing myself to be twenty pounds underweight. Also, my husband was very instrumental in my change of thinking—he loved me and helped boost my self-esteem. I quit performing and started teaching dance instead. Ever since then, I've maintained a healthy weight, but I never got over not wanting breasts. I always felt that the larger they were, the heavier I looked. So when I decided to have a prophylactic mastectomy, I wasn't tormented over 'losing' my breasts. To me, they were just pieces of fat on my body."

While Suzanne had only negative thoughts of her breasts, there are women like Lisa, Mayde, and Amy, who were always somewhat neutral about them. "My breasts served a purpose with breast-feeding and they looked fine in clothes, but they were never a big part of my identity," explains Mayde.

And, of course, plenty of women view their breasts as a defining part of their sexuality. Rori says hers were always an important part of who she was. "I remember when I was in the fifth grade, I hadn't developed yet but my chest was starting to feel very sore," she recalls. "I would press down on it and the pain was severe. But I didn't care because I wanted boobs. I saw how much my mom and older sisters loved their breasts, and I longed to have them myself. Nothing happened right away, but I waited patiently and begged my mom to take me shopping for my first training bra. I was envious of my girlfriends who had already started to develop. I couldn't wait.

"I was in seventh or eighth grade when it happened," Rori continues. "I finally started to have breasts. And they were great! I don't even remember them growing in stages. I had these little tiny buds and then—va-va-voom. I was so happy.

"By the time I was in ninth grade, I was a 36C. My friends thought I was so lucky, but then I started getting a lot of attention from the boys, which made me uncomfortable. It seemed like they never looked up to see my face. It angered me. I went through a period where I was so tired of getting attention from my breasts that I even considered having a breast reduction. But luckily I never got one because after I married my high school sweetheart and had three kids, I began to really appreciate my breasts more than ever. My mother always told me that the feeling you get from breast-feeding is indescribable. I know it's not like that for everyone, but for me it was an amazing experience. From that point on, I truly loved my breasts—they were a huge part of my confidence, my sexuality, and how I dressed. I liked the way they looked and how it felt when my husband or I touched them. So the very thought of having mine altered in any way was nearly impossible to swallow."

"boca boobs"

Lisa, Mayde, Amy, Rori, and Suzanne all live in or near Boca Raton, Florida. Breast enhancement surgery is so common in that part of the country that Mayde and her daughter, Phoebe, play a game in the mall where they whisper "Boob alert" when they see a woman with obviously fake breasts. The game keeps them quite busy—along with Southern California and Texas, South Florida is where women opt for the biggest implants, says Mark Pinsky, M.D., a plastic surgeon in Palm Beach and spokesperson for Allergan, a leading implant manufacturer. Also, because of the temperate year-round climate, women in Florida tend to wear more revealing clothing, regardless of whether their breasts are real or not.

So when these five women were deciding to have reconstruction with implants after their mastectomies, it was important to them that their results didn't look obvious. "For me, the whole vision of getting implants was, 'Oh my God, I'm going to wind up with the stereotypical Boca boobs,'" says Mayde. "That's not what I wanted. I didn't want round enormous melons. I didn't want to look fake."

Amy says she doesn't even consider her operation in the same category. "I never put myself in the same league as women who have breast augmentation," she says. "They haven't lost feeling in their breasts. And they didn't have their surgeries out of fear of cancer."

Because they live in such a breast-conscious society, these women experienced some shocking reactions from people after they had their surgeries. Lisa in particular still can't get over some of the comments she heard. "I'll never forgot this one acquaintance who came up to me in the gym and said, 'Welcome to the club,' meaning the 'club' of women who had gotten breast implants," she recalls. "All I could think was, 'Are you kidding me? Maybe I'm in a prophylactic mastectomy club, but I'm certainly not in the same club as you. I didn't do this because I wanted bigger breasts. I watched my mother die from breast cancer. I did this to avoid following in her footsteps.'"

Suzanne also found it shocking that some people were jealous that she had the surgery. "They'd actually say, 'You're so lucky. I want to say I have a family history of breast cancer so I can justify getting my boobs done,'" she recalls. "I'd think, 'You may feel that way, but, trust me, you don't want to trade places with me. I'm sure you'd take flat-chested with no risk over beautiful breasts and BRCA2 any day.'"

And it's not only other women who seem to miss the big picture—many men don't realize that a prophylactic mastectomy is a far cry from a "boob job." Lisa says that some people were so curious about her new breasts that they'd stare at her chest, though the last thing she wanted from this surgery was extra attention. One friend's husband took it a step further. "We went out with another couple for dinner, and while the four of us were sitting at the table the man motioned toward my chest and jokingly said, 'Hey Lisa, they're looking good. Maybe you can let me see them later,'" Lisa recalls. "Then he turned to my husband, Bob, and said, 'How do you like them?' It was like he was buying a car and he wanted to go for a test drive. He kept cracking jokes like that and he and his wife couldn't stop laughing. But this wasn't a joke for me."

Lisa says that she believes that if someone wants to undergo breast augmentation, that's her prerogative. But what bothers her is that women getting implants don't seem to experience nearly half the backlash that women having prophylactic mastectomies might. "Implants are a dime a dozen these days and society only seems to encourage breast enhancement surgery," Lisa says. "So what's with the controversy over having a surgery that has a similar end result but also may save my life? If these women can do it, why can't I?"

choosing new breasts

If you opt to have a prophylactic mastectomy, don't be surprised if you and everyone around you become more preoccupied with the final appearance of your breasts than with the surgery itself. It can be a complicated decision, one that each woman will approach differently. "Post-mastectomy reconstruction patients are looking to feel 'normal' again, but their needs vary greatly," says Anthony Dardano, D.O., a plastic surgeon and chief of surgery at Boca Raton Community

Hospital. "Some women simply want a mound to fill a bra. Others want their surgeon to re-create the same breasts they had. And then there are those who want to make the most out of this opportunity and try to improve their appearance."

Typically, when a woman first visits her plastic surgeon, he'll measure her bust and possibly show her pictures of patients with different breast sizes to get an idea of what her desires are. Also, the doctor might ask, "Do you want to be bigger or smaller? Would you like to be perkier? Are you hoping for a natural look? Do you want to fix any imperfections (some you might not have even known you had)?"

Here are some terms you might want to be familiar with when you have such conversations:

Volume: The weight of the implant in cubic centimeters (cc's). After the mastectomy, your surgeon may weigh the tissue he has removed from your breast. The weight in grams is about the equivalent to its weight in cc's. Some experts estimate that roughly every 150 to 200 cc's equals a cup size.

Profile: A lot of times women don't necessarily want their breasts to be bigger. They just want them to be perkier. That's where profile comes into play—it's the distance the implants project off the chest wall. Typically, there are three choices: low, moderate, and high. (Some implant manufacturers might have different names for these options. For instance, Mentor offers moderate, moderate plus, and high.) The higher the category, the more the projection.

Shape: Round or shaped (there are many different-shaped varieties, such as teardrop or contoured).

Texture: Smooth or textured surface. Some experts prefer using textured implants because they are less likely to cause capsular contraction (where the tissue that forms around the implants tightens, possibly making them feel very firm and look distorted). However, textured implants can be more visible through the skin and more prone to wrinkling. Shaped implants are almost always textured so that they stay in place—if a round implant moves, it's still round, but if a shaped implant moves, the result can look awkward.

Cohesiveness: Refers to the material that fills an implant. Saline implants contain a saltwater solution. Silicone implants are filled with gel, though they vary in density and cohesiveness.

Skin envelope: The amount and elasticity of the skin remaining after a mastectomy is crucial when determining implant size and shape (and, in some cases, whether or not a woman can keep her nipple). A woman who is overweight and has breast-fed three children might have enough skin to accommodate a considerably larger implant than her original breast size. In fact, rippling or wrinkling can occur when a doctor doesn't completely fill the skin envelope after surgery. On the flip side, another woman with little skin left might not have tissue that will stretch to accommodate a large implant.

Expanders: Women and their surgeons sometimes opt for expanders either because there is not enough skin to accommodate an implant, or they want to get a better idea of what size the woman's breasts will be after surgery. Through a port in the skin, the doctor fills the expander with a saline solution, stretching the skin and muscle until a woman is happy with the way her chest looks. He then removes the expander and, in a second surgery, swaps it out with a permanent implant that's the same size.

Flap surgeries: As far as flap surgeries are concerned, the size of your new breasts will be dependent on the amount of fat layer you have in your body. For instance, if you want a TRAM surgery that takes fat from your stomach, but you have a tummy only the size of a B cup, then a B cup is the biggest you can go. If you opt to go bigger, you'll need to choose either implants or a flap and implant combination surgery.

Some women are very involved in the process of choosing their new breasts. When Lisa was making that decision, for example, she went to a doctor in her hometown to try on implants. She brought along different bras and shirts to get a good idea of how various sizes looked on her body. She also spent hours searching websites where you can compare yourself with other women on the basis of height, weight, and measurements. Even her husband helped out. "It was like we were shopping for new breasts," Lisa says.

Other women aren't that involved at all. Mayde, for instance, simply brought in a picture of Heather Locklear as her ideal and told her doctor she didn't want it to be obvious she had had surgery. Amy had a similar experience. "I went for my consultation and my surgeon's nurse brought me into a room to show me before-and-after pictures of people who had had the same surgery I was having," she says. "I had a hard time envisioning what I would look like, so I just said, 'I just want to be me.'"

Either way, many women ultimately put their fate in the hands of their doctor which, of course, you should do only if you've found a reputable one (see Chapter 9). That way you don't have to drive yourself crazy trying to figure out cc's and all the other particulars of your implants. Instead, you can get a general idea of what you like and then trust your surgeon. For that reason, Suzanne says she went from a small A cup to a full B. "I had issues with the larger size, but my doctor said that when you empty the skin pocket and don't fill it enough, you can get wrinkling because of the excess skin," Suzanne explains. "Actually, that happened to Rori, and right before my surgery she said, 'Listen to Dr. Salzberg,' who was doctor for both of us. So I did, and thankfully Rori was right."

Adds Mark Pinsky, M.D., a plastic surgeon in Palm Beach, "Keep in mind that when choosing an implant, many factors need to be taken into consideration, such as a patient's weight, the width of her chest and breast, the elasticity of the breast tissue, whether or not she's small or big boned, and the patient's goals. It's not as simple as picking out an A, B, C, or D cup. That's why it's crucial that a woman has a back-and-forth dialogue with her surgeon about what she desires and what's attainable. Ultimately, the most important element is that the dimension of the implant matches the proportion of a woman's figure."

is bigger better?

Regardless of what size you choose, chances are other people are going to have an opinion about the "new you." Mayde says she has a friend with enormous implants who wears tight T-shirts and no bra. She loves the attention. So when Mayde showed this woman her results, her friend was flabbergasted. "She told me, 'You're crazy. You're too small. You should have gone bigger,'" Mayde recalls. "I said, 'No, I wanted to feel as natural as possible.' She just kept shaking her head like I was nuts. She couldn't understand why anyone wouldn't choose breasts like hers. But this wasn't about size for me. It was about reducing my risk of developing breast cancer."

Lisa also felt a lot of pressure. "When I went to test out implants, the doctor's nurse kept putting in ones that were so enormous," she says. "One was the size and weight of a large grapefruit." Even Lisa's classy, conservative, nearly seventy-year-old friend, whom she brought along for help, surprised Lisa when she said, "Honey, go as big as you can. You have one chance to get it right." "I was going for a natural look, but I kept getting bombarded with the message 'Bigger is better,'" says Lisa. "Celebrities in magazines, movies, and even these women made me question my smaller breasts."

BODY IMAGE

Regardless of how a woman opts to confront her breast cancer risk, her decision can certainly take a toll on her both psychologically and emotionally. Body image is one such issue women most commonly report. Here's why:

Body Image and Surveillance

While increased surveillance might not have as much of an effect on body image as a mastectomy might, it *can* affect how a woman views her breasts. For instance, a woman who has spent years fearing every mammogram, ultrasound, or MRI might start resenting her breasts for bringing such stress into her life. Also, when a person has undergone multiple biopsies, the scars can affect her opinion of her appearance. For instance, Mayde says that her multiple biopsies left her feeling that her breasts were being "chipped away" bit by bit. And Lisa adds that she hates the scars on her chest—ironically, *not* the ones from her mastectomy, which are hidden underneath the fold of her breasts, but the ones she got when she had several suspicious lumps removed years ago.

Body Image and Chemoprevention

Many women don't want to try chemoprevention as a risk-reducing option because they're afraid of the side effects. Taking tamoxifen can lead to vaginal dryness, vaginal discharge, hot flashes, fatigue, and bladder problems. The most common side effects of raloxifene include hot flashes, swelling, sweating, leg cramps, joint pain, and flu-like symptoms. Though no studies have shown that tamoxifen or raloxifene cause weight gain, anecdotally many women say that they do.

In fact, experts report that very few women offered tamoxifen or raloxifene for chemoprevention take the drugs, mostly because they're afraid of hot flashes, fatigue, and weight gain. And Mayde remembers asking a leading breast surgeon in New York why so many high-risk women don't choose chemoprevention. He told her that once women heard that they might gain weight, they knocked that option off the list.

Body Image After a Mastectomy

While having a prophylactic mastectomy is difficult on many levels, one of the most trying aspects is how a woman feels about her body after the surgery. Body image is a main reason many women elect not to go through with it, says Marlene Frost, R.N., Ph.D., who conducts patient-reported outcome research at the Mayo Clinic Women's Cancer Program in Minnesota. Some women say they feel like they'd lose a part of their sexuality and an essential aspect of their femininity. Rori can relate. She says that if the nipple-sparing procedure she had hadn't been an option—a surgery that left the appearance of her breasts nearly intact—she would have continued with surveillance.

Other women actually report that their body image is better than ever after their surgeries. "For some women who have been worried about breast cancer their whole lives, this operation can relieve so much anxiety that they feel like they have a new lease on life," says Jennifer Klemp, Ph.D., a psychologist and cancer risk counselor at the University of Kansas Breast Cancer Prevention Center.

That was the case for Lisa. "I sometimes resented my breasts because they brought me a lot of pain and heartache, and I was constantly worried that something was happening inside of them," she says. "After my surgery, a great weight was lifted off of me because I had finally gotten rid of most of my risk. It wasn't that the appearance of my breasts improved greatly. For me, I just felt healthier overall, and that translated to a better body image."

Suzanne agrees that eliminating danger was a huge positive factor. "I had always considered my breasts these lethal things waiting to kill me, so my perception of them improved dramatically," she says. She adds that she finally started to like their appearance, too. "My breasts were always kind of small and they had an odd shape, so now I think I look nicer in clothes and I feel more womanly," she says. "That's not why I had the surgery, but it was certainly a nice benefit." Mayde, too, was pleased with her results. "The reconstruction after my mastectomy helped make my deflated, post-nursing, aging breasts a little perkier," she says. "I feel great."

While most women don't regret having prophylactic mastectomies, some do have a difficult time dealing with their cosmetic results. Ultimately, some women are going to have body image issues, especially those who have struggled with body image their whole life, experts say. In fact, a study in the *Journal of Clinical Oncology* found that when women who had prophylactic mastectomies were surveyed one year after their surgeries, about half of them reported a negative impact on sexuality and body image. The women in this study said that they felt more insecure about their appearance, less sexually attractive, and unhappy with scars. Dr. Frost from the Mayo Clinic also found in her research that satisfaction with body image, feelings of femininity, and sexual relationships were the most negatively affected psychological or social variables after women had contralateral prophylactic mastectomies.

Amy, for instance, says, "I'm happy I had my surgery, but I have felt less whole at times." And Joy Larsen Haidle, a genetic counselor at the Humphrey Cancer Center in Minnesota adds, "Many women take a long time to come to grips with the fact that 'this is the new me.' Some say they feel grief when they look at their chest after the surgery. That sense of loss is real."

That's particularly true when a woman has complications. Rori says that after her mastectomy, she had a very difficult time adjusting to her new breasts. "Once I healed, I had a dent in one breast and rippling and sagging," she says. "I looked fine in clothes, but when I took them off I didn't like the way my breasts looked. So, two years after my first operation, I went back to New York for a revision. It was so stressful having to deal with the financial, emotional, and physical impact of the surgery again, but I was so unhappy that I knew I'd regret it if I didn't try for a better outcome. And I'm thrilled that I did—I love the way my breasts look now."

Some women have much worse initial reactions than Rori had. On some message boards women talk about feeling "ugly," "unattractive," and crushed by their results. They say they're "disgusted" by the way they look, and they have "overwhelming feelings of regret" about how their body turned out. Many complain of scars and complications and make comments like "I can't look at myself in the mirror," and "I can't stop crying."

Suzanne in particular remembers one woman who had had her nipples removed said, "I look like a Barbie doll with a zipper across my chest." Suzanne says, "I'd read stories like this and I'd think, 'What am I getting myself into?' But thankfully I had met Mayde that fateful day at my dance studio. She was there for me from when I first started confronting my risk through my surgery and beyond. So when I'd hear horror stories about surgeries gone wrong, Mayde would talk me off the ledge by saying, 'Stop making yourself crazy. Worrying is a waste of time. You're going to be fine.' Mayde was so upbeat and kept reassuring me that she was thrilled with her results. I knew that not everyone felt the same way as she did, but I figured I just had to believe that those negative things weren't going to happen to me. I kept reminding myself that even if my cosmetic outcome was far from perfect, it couldn't be as bad as having breast cancer."

Also, it's important to note that sometimes doing research *before* the surgery can help prevent feelings of disappointment afterward. As discussed in Chapter 9, taking steps like making sure you find the right surgeon, seeing before-and-after pictures of previous patients, and talking to other women who have already had their mastectomies can prepare you emotionally and physically. Not all of the women in this book would say that their mastectomy results were flawless or that their recoveries were a breeze. However, they weren't devastated because they had set realistic expectations (as explained at the end of this chapter).

body image after an oophorectomy

While removing ovaries doesn't affect a woman's outward appearance, the loss of hormones produced by the ovaries can lead to menopausal symptoms such as vaginal dryness, loss of sexual libido, mood changes, dry skin, and hot flashes (not to mention a higher risk for osteoporosis and heart disease). Also, many women have a difficult time dealing not just with the loss of their fertility, but with what it means symbolically as well. Some women believe that their ovaries and ability to have babies is what makes them different from men. To them, an oophorectomy not only removes those organs, but also eliminates their female identity.

Though no definitive study has shown that premature menopause will affect a woman's metabolism, some women say their greatest fear is gaining weight. Suzanne says that's one of the main reasons she hasn't had an oophorectomy yet, even though she knows her risk of ovarian cancer is way above average. "I know it's inevitable that someday I'll face menopause, but I don't want to be dealing with it in my forties," she says. "Considering all of the body issues I've faced in the past, I'm petrified I'll gain weight and age prematurely. I know that if I were talking to someone battling ovarian cancer, my comments would seem shallow to her. She would think, 'You're worried about gaining a few pounds and I'm dying here. Are you crazy?' But I admit it. That's a huge reason why I keep putting off the surgery."

Rori says she was also afraid of having her ovaries removed, but because of the prevalence of ovarian cancer in her family, she felt like she had no choice but to have the surgery. And after the operation, initially she was miserable. "I had no sex drive, horrible hot flashes, and vaginal dryness," says Rori. "All I could think was, 'I'm only thirty-eight years old. I hope I didn't make a mistake.' But eventually, I found the right hormone replacement therapy for me (bioidentical hormones) and now those symptoms are under control."

Of course, not all women experience only negative side effects after having their ovaries removed. Rori says that, in many ways, having the surgery wound up changing her for the better. "When I used to get my period, I'd have mood swings, painful cysts, and such awful cramps that I'd have to stay home in bed for a few days, taking Motrin," she says. "My breasts were so tender I couldn't touch them. And between the bloating and my giving in to every craving, I'd feel fat and disgusting. However, ever since my surgery, I have felt one hundred times better in my body. I don't have the hormonal ups and downs I used to have, and I feel more even keel overall."

the importance of expectations

Dealing with the aftermath of risk-reducing options is never easy. But experts say one of the best ways to prevent disappointment is by setting realistic expectations and doing your homework. "I always tell my patients that, when it comes to prophylactic mastectomies, they should ask to see pictures of their surgeons' best and worst results," says Jennifer Klemp, Ph.D., a psychologist and cancer risk counselor at the University of Kansas Breast Cancer Prevention Center. "I want a woman to know she might not have an amazing cosmetic outcome. She might wind up with scars, have complications, or lose most of the sensation in her breasts. Some people go in thinking none of these things are possible, and they're the ones who are more likely to be dissatisfied afterward."

One solution is for doctors to make more of an effort when it comes to understanding a woman's expectations *before* she has a prophylactic surgery. "Women having this operation are a very different patient group from those with an actual cancer diagnosis," says Andrea Pusic, M.D., a plastic surgeon at Memorial Sloan-Kettering Cancer Center in New York City. "They may have much higher expectations of what their results will be after reconstruction." For that reason, Dr. Pusic spearheaded the development of BREAST-Q, a questionnaire for women who have had mastectomies and/or reconstruction, among other breast surgeries. Doctors both nationally and internationally can use the questionnaire to gauge their patients' satisfaction with the surgical process and contentment with the outcome. The purpose? "As doctors, we can achieve higher patient satisfaction if we consistently measure and address their expectations preoperatively," says Dr. Pusic. "When we don't, then no matter what technique we're using or how well the surgery goes, if a patient's expectations were something different, she'll be dissatisfied and the outcome will affect her quality of life."

Other experts also stress the importance of taking steps to fight your risk only when you're ready. They say that women who take their time weighing the options are much happier than women who make hasty decisions. Of course, a woman's threshold of what results she's willing to live with is completely individual. Women need to gather all the information they can, whether it be about surveillance, tamoxifen or raloxifene, or a prophylactic surgery they plan to have. They should know why some women are unhappy afterward, and then they can determine if they could live with those results.

Rori says she understands this strategy all too well. "When I was preparing for my mastectomy, I read everything I could about any complications that might happen," she says. "I also asked my doctor to see before-and-after pictures (something many surgeons and online sources provide), even ones that showed women bruising while they healed. I was confident about my decision to have my operation, but I wasn't going in blind. And though I eventually felt unhappy with my cosmetic result, my preparation made it easier for me to deal with it because I knew rippling and wrinkling was a possibility. I had gone ahead with the surgery anyway because nothing was more important to me than lowering my risk of breast cancer. So despite the fact that I didn't love my results at first, I felt lucky that I accomplished what I set out to do."

CHAPTER TWELVE

the hidden killer in men

Lisa's grandfather, Lou, may have had a secret that not even he knew. And it potentially led to the death of his own daughter—Lisa's mother, Arlene. "When my grandfather wound up in the hospital right before he died, the doctors discovered a golf ball–sized lump on his chest," Lisa says. "I remember seeing it and thinking it was so big. It turned out he had breast cancer, but for some reason, knowing that didn't translate to my mom being more vigilant. Unfortunately, there was no blood test for the BRCA gene mutations back then. But when my mother later tested positive for BRCA2, it was pretty obvious that it was my grandfather who passed it to her because my grandmother didn't have any breast or ovarian cancer in her family."

Many people falsely believe that a woman can inherit a risk for breast cancer only from her mother's side of the family. That's simply not true—men are just as likely to carry BRCA gene mutations as women are. And when they do, it can have serious health implications for them as well as their families (though a man's risk of developing breast cancer still isn't remotely as great as it is for a woman). If a man has one of these mutations, that means not only that he's at increased risk for certain cancers, but also that his daughters may have a very significant chance of developing breast and/or ovarian cancers if they inherit the mutation from him. "For a long time, many experts didn't realize that when it came to breast cancer we needed to look at both the mother's *and* father's history," explains Victor Vogel, M.D., national vice president of research for the American Cancer Society. "Now we know that we do."

a red flag

Breast cancer is an equal opportunity disease—it affects people of all religions, ethnicities, and ages. And though approximately 99 percent of people affected are women, men are not without risk. In fact, according to the American Cancer Society, almost two thousand men are diagnosed with breast cancer each year. Because it's so rare for a man to have breast cancer, it's a major warning sign that there's a BRCA gene mutation in the family. And that's something Lisa and her family wish they had known. "We had no idea that the tumor on my grandfather's chest was an indication that we were in danger," Lisa says. "My mother's doctor never said anything to her like 'Oh my God. Your father had breast cancer. You're at risk.' His attitude was more like 'Your father had a tumor and died,' but he never said whether or not that affected her. He even put my mom on hormone replacement therapy, which was a big mistake, because it was adding estrogen to her body. No doctor ever even mentioned that my grandfather's breast cancer might increase my mother's risk of the disease until my mom had already been diagnosed with it and the two of us went to see a genetics expert. When we told that expert about my grandfather, she explained that his breast cancer was a red flag that there is a genetic mutation in our family. She said there was no question we should undergo testing. Unfortunately, we found that out when it was already too late for my mom."

It's critical to remember that, as is the case with women, a man can have a mutated BRCA1 or BRCA2 gene and never develop cancer at all. However, he *can* pass that gene on to his children. It's like a flip of a coin—if a man is BRCA-positive, there's a 50/50 chance that each of his children will be, too. Many men who understand this concept and choose to get tested say they're doing so only for their daughters. But plenty don't go down that road, and that's a major concern, because when this gene mutation becomes hidden—or, in other words, a man never learns he has it—his children and grandchildren might never know they're at risk until they're facing the unthinkable. Mayde has seen this happen. "I have a friend who was diagnosed with breast cancer when she was thirty-six and then tested positive for BRCA," Mayde says. "She knew some women in her dad's family had had breast cancer, but she never thought she was at risk. When my friend learned that she probably inherited the mutation from her dad, she was floored. Who would have thought you could inherit the breast cancer gene from your father?"

Dr. Vogel says the key to protecting yourself is to learn about any cancers on both your mother's *and* father's side. He once had a female patient with breast cancer who tested negative for a BRCA mutation. That woman's husband decided to get tested, too, because there were several cases of breast cancer in his family. It turned out *he* was positive. "This couple's daughters thought they were in the clear when their mom tested negative, but they actually wound up inheriting the gene from their dad," says Dr. Vogel. "I consider them lucky for finding out about their risk before something terrible happened. We would have missed it completely if we had just focused on their mother."

The signs that indicate a man might have a genetic mutation are the same as they are for a woman. For instance, a man may want to consider getting genetic counseling and possibly testing if any of the following are in his family:

- A known BRCA mutation.
- Any ovarian cancer or male breast cancer.

- Any relative with two cases of cancer (e.g., breast and ovarian, or two different breast cancers).
- Any breast cancer and an Ashkenazi Jewish heritage.
- Multiple cases of breast and/or ovarian cancer, especially in people younger than fifty.

consequences of brca in men

When a man carries a BRCA2 gene mutation, he has significantly higher odds for developing certain cancers than the average man. For some reason, BRCA1 mutations in men don't seem to affect their risk much (though it *can* affect their children). Here's a breakdown of how a man's risk is affected:

Prostate cancer: This disease is the number-one non-skin cancer among men—about 192,000 men in the United States developed it in 2009. However, while the average man has a one-in-six chance of being diagnosed with this cancer during his lifetime, those with a BRCA2 mutation may have as high as a one-in-three risk. Also, most cases of prostate cancer occur in men older than sixty-five. But when a man has a BRCA gene mutation, this disease often manifests earlier.

Breast cancer: Although breast cancer is rare in men, those men who have BRCA mutations carry a greater risk for the disease than men who don't. Whereas the average man's risk of developing breast cancer in his lifetime is less than 0.1 percent, the chances are 1.2 percent for male BRCA1 mutation carriers and 6.8 percent for men with a BRCA2 mutation, per a study in the *Journal of the National Cancer Institute*.

Other cancers: According to the American Cancer Society, other cancers have been associated with BRCA mutations in men, such as pancreatic cancer, melanoma, and cancers of the stomach. These cancers may develop at a younger age than they would in men in the general population. However, keep in mind that even with BRCA mutations, a man's risk for many of these cancers is still low and pales in comparison with the breast and ovarian cancer risk a woman with either mutation faces.

the reluctance to test

Despite all the reasons that men should face their risk, sometimes persuading them to get tested is easier said than done. The main reason they may be hesitant to do so is that they think of BRCA as a women's issue, one that just doesn't pertain to them, experts say. In fact, one study found that the majority of men are unaware of their risk and consequently few want to get tested. "A lot of what motivates people to take measures to protect their health is their perceived risk," explains Paul Jacobsen, Ph.D., chair of health outcomes and behavior at Moffitt Cancer Center in Tampa. "The problem is, with BRCA, men just don't think they're susceptible. They also don't quite understand that they can inherit a genetic mutation and pass it on to their children."

Suzanne has witnessed this attitude firsthand. "I have six male cousins on my mom's side, and though all of them have a very good chance of having the BRCA2 mutation that's in our family, none have gotten tested," she says. "The scary part is that all of them have daughters who range in age from fifteen to thirty and might have inherited their risk from them. The only reason I can imagine my cousins won't get tested is because they don't fully understand what having this mutation means. I tried talking to them, but they don't want to hear it. Their reactions have been along the lines of 'Why are you making such a big deal out of this? I don't have breasts, so what do I need to know this for?' It's like they're in denial. I'm hoping a news report or something will get their attention, but if not, I'll take it upon myself to inform their daughters when the time is right. What pisses me off is that my cousins haven't done their homework. If they sought genetic counseling and then decided not to get tested, fine. But I don't understand how they can make a decision without being informed. What if, God forbid, one of their kids gets breast or ovarian cancer? I feel like they're playing Russian roulette with their children's lives."

Often, even when men do understand their risk, they don't want to get tested because they don't see the point in doing so. Rori says one of her cousins who doesn't have children and another cousin who has two boys will not get tested. "They both have the attitude, 'If I get cancer, *then* I'll deal with it,'" she says. There are also men who figure they'll avoid the test altogether and let their daughters take it if they want to, or they'll wait until their children are older to get tested. Amy's brother, for instance, was going to take the test, but he changed his mind. "My brother's daughter is only seven, so it's not like she can get tested or do anything preventatively at this point," Amy says. "My brother isn't in a huge rush to get tested because she's so young."

One of Lisa's brothers feels the same way. He went for genetic counseling but never followed up with the test even though their mother had the BRCA2 mutation. "He keeps telling me excuses like 'I have new insurance' or 'I've been busy,' but I think deep down he figures he'll face all of this when his daughters are older and he feels like he *has* to," Lisa says. However, what worries Lisa is that her other brother doesn't want to get tested at all. He has three sons and does all the recommended screening for cancers that he may have an increased risk to develop, so he thinks there's no point in him knowing. "What's frightening," says Lisa, "is that if he never tells his sons they might be at risk, those boys could be positive for BRCA2 and never know it. Then, if someday they have daughters, they can pass the mutation on to them. That's how this gene hides itself—just like it did with my grandfather."

taking steps

Men who know they carry a BRCA gene mutation can help protect themselves by being screened regularly for some of the cancers for which they might be at an increased risk. For prostate cancer, experts suggest that men talk to their doctor about whether they should start getting their annual PSA (prostate-specific antigen) blood test and digital exam at an earlier age than fifty. Because male breast cancer is so rare, there is no national recommendation for screening mammography. Instead, men should see a doctor if there are any lumps or changes in their breast tissue. Experts also suggest they have annual screenings for melanoma. Of course, exercising, limiting alcohol, and maintaining a healthy weight can't hurt—such lifestyle changes have been shown to decrease the odds of many cancers.

If there's a man in your life who should be following these screening suggestions or considering genetic counseling or testing, you might want to encourage him to do so. Research shows he might not do it on his own—according to the National Center for Health Statistics, women are much more likely than men to seek medical care of any kind. While ultimately it's his decision, the best way to help a man you care about is by arming him with the information he needs to make the best choice for him. For instance, offer to make him an appointment with a genetic counselor, or e-mail him links to articles about the cancer risks for men and their offspring associated with BRCA mutations. (The American Cancer Society website, for one, offers helpful information.)

Suzanne is grateful that her brother finally decided to take action.

"At first, when I told my brother, who has two daughters, about getting tested, his reaction was, 'Why would I want to do this?'" she recalls. "But then I gave him sources for learning more about BRCA. I also told him, 'If you test negative, then your daughters won't have to worry. But if you test positive, then you could have possibly passed this gene on to them, and that's information they deserve to know.' He agreed and, for his daughters' sakes, decided to get tested. My brother tested positive for BRCA2. Next, my nieces tested—one was negative, the other was positive and has since had a prophylactic mastectomy. I'm really proud of my brother for dealing with this difficult issue. I think he ultimately gave a gift to his daughters."

a mother's legacy

When Amy first began facing her breast cancer risk, she says her kids were all she could think about. "During that time, I'd sneak into my daughter Marley's room at night to check on her and I'd start to cry," she recalls. "I would just stare at her and pray, 'Please, don't let her go through what I'm going through.' To this day, I'd hate to think that her breasts might ever cause her the fear that mine have caused me."

While dealing with any of the issues related to breast cancer risk can be complicated and confusing, being a mother adds an extra layer of fear, guilt, worry, and motivation to the mix. Rori says that with every decision she made about her risk, her first thoughts were: "How is this going to affect my children? What should I tell them? Will they someday have to face these same issues?" Whether you're a mother of a toddler, a teenager, or a grown adult, chances are you might be grappling with some of these same thoughts and concerns.

a major motivator

For many women, being a mother fuels most decisions they make in their lives. And there's no exception when it comes to their dealing with their health. "Women take a lot of factors into consideration when facing their cancer risk, and one of those is how they perceive they're needed by their children or loved ones," says Talia Donenberg, a genetic counselor at the University of Miami/Sylvester Comprehensive Cancer Center. "Parents tend to be more aggressive in choosing risk-reducing strategies because their main goal is making sure they're around for their kids."

Suzanne agrees that her daughter, Nina, was her number one motivator. "All I could think was that I have to be there for my child, who was only seven at the time of my surgery," she says. "That motherly instinct is what made me go into the operating room for my mastectomy. I grew up without my mom—she died when I was only four—and if there was anything in my power to prevent Nina from sharing the same fate, I'd do it." Lisa adds that the memory of watching her mother, Arlene, die is what persuaded her to schedule her surgery. "Seeing my mom suffer and then losing her was the worst thing that ever happened to me," she says. "I wasn't going to let my kids experience that same kind of pain if I could help it."

Rori also says she felt a sense of responsibility to her daughter, Jensen, and two sons, Ryland and Linden. "When I decided to get genetic testing, I knew I had to be prepared to deal with the outcome," she says. "Knowing I have such a high risk for breast and ovarian cancer, how could I not at least do surveillance? If I didn't have kids, fine. But I brought these people into the world, and I have a moral obligation to them. I'm not going to let them lose me because of something I could have prevented."

Many women and men also say that being a parent or grandparent is why they got tested in the first place. They wanted to know if they carried a BRCA gene mutation so they could pass that knowledge on to their children and grandchildren. Amy explains, "Of course I wanted to get tested to find out my own risk, but I also wanted to know what cards I might have dealt my kids. I was more worried about them than I was about myself."

As for Mayde, she was motivated not only by her two children and the memories of her mother's battle with breast cancer, but also by the stories of other mothers who had the disease. "After I found out that I had LCIS and ADH, conditions which indicated I had a greater chance of developing invasive cancer down the road, I thought back to a post I once read on the FORCE message board," Mayde recalls. "A woman with metastasized breast cancer said her doctor had told her she had three more months to live. That woman's response was something along the lines of 'How can I have only three more months when I need thirty more years to be with my children?' Her quote left such an impact on me. So when I was deciding how to deal with my own risk, I wasn't thinking about myself. All I could think about were these two little lives I had to care for, and that I needed to stick around for a very long time."

talking to your kids about risk

Discussing breast cancer risk with children can be a difficult task—it's a complicated topic that many adults don't even understand. Experts say that it's important to talk about this issue with your kids when you think they're ready—many suggest eighteen or older as an appropriate age. However, researchers at Fox Chase Cancer Center and the University of Chicago found that about half of parents with a BRCA mutation told their minor children about it.

There are possible pros and cons of having such a discussion with children or adolescents, says Angela Bradbury, M.D., lead author of the study and director of the Margaret Dyson Family Risk Assessment Program at Fox Chase Cancer Center in Philadelphia. On the one hand, half of the parents who told their children about the BRCA mutation in the family reported that their kids were initially anxious or frightened by the news. On the other hand, further data suggest that children who learn there is such a mutation in their family may adopt healthier behaviors because of their possible risk. For instance, some of the older offspring quit smoking, started eating better, or exercising more, says Dr. Bradbury. It's important, she adds, to decide on a case-by-case basis whether you think your child can handle such potent news. Also, talk to your kids' doctors about whether or not your children should take preventative measures just in case they do have a BRCA mutation. For instance, you might want to discuss limiting the number of X-rays they get, and whether or not they should avoid taking oral contraceptives.

In terms of what to say when you *do* decide to discuss risk with your son or daughter, here are the main principles: Keep it simple, be honest, and always be prepared to answer questions. Amy says that while it won't be easy, she plans to be open with her kids, Ryan, Marley, and Dylan, about their potential risk. "My children are too young to talk about the BRCA gene, but I'll definitely have that conversation with them when they either ask me about it or when I feel the time is right," she says. "I would never want them to turn to me one day and say, 'You never told me about this.'"

Sometimes teens will ask whether or not they need to get tested. Again, that's an area up for debate. Most experts agree that people shouldn't be tested until they're *at least* eighteen years old. However, many parents want to know if they've passed a BRCA mutation on to their kids sooner rather than later. Some news accounts tell of children as young as four getting tested. "When a mother or father tests positive for a BRCA mutation, one of the most common things they struggle with is that they want to know as soon as possible that their kids are negative," explains Joy Larsen Haidle, a genetic counselor at the Humphrey Cancer Center in Minnesota. She adds that she believes it's important not to take away your child's right *not* to test. "While you want to know the result is negative so you can move on with your lives, what if it's positive?" says Larsen Haidle. "How would you handle knowing such news when your child is, say, ten, but you can't do anything about it [let alone discuss it] for years?"

Ever the optimist, Rori says she barely thinks about the possibility that her kids carry the genetic mutation she has. "There's no point in worrying about something that we won't have to face for years," she says. "Until then, I want my kids to live healthy, complete, carefree lives. I don't want their potential risk for cancer to affect their paths in life. And if and when the time comes that they have to deal with their risk, I'll support them with whatever they want to do. But I just figure there might be much better options for them than there were for me, so what's the use in getting worked up about their choices now?"

On the other hand, Amy says the very thought that her kids, particularly her daughter, Marley, might have a BRCA mutation weighs heavily on her mind. "Part of me really wants them to get tested now," she says. "But, even more so, I want my kids to take that step when the time is right for them. In a perfect world, I'd love for my daughter to be married and have kids and then get tested like I did. But I know that she will make the choice when she's ready."

Since Lisa and Mayde both tested negative, their children's risk for breast cancer is either similar to that of the general population or slightly greater because of their family history, depending on which expert you ask. Lisa says that she's relieved her children won't have a BRCA mutation, but she says she'll always want to make sure they keep on top of their health. Her daughter Emmy is seven and still a bit young to initiate conversations about risk. However, her older daughter, Gabby, who's now thirteen, does the initiating herself. "Gabby often asks me if she's at risk," Lisa explains. "We didn't tell her that my mother was battling breast cancer until right before my mom died, so maybe Gabby doesn't trust me when I tell her that she's going to be okay. Even so, I still want my children to always feel comfortable talking to me about any health concerns or issues."

Mayde agrees and adds that she hopes her whole experience is a lesson for her children. "Even though I won't pass on a genetic mutation to them because I tested negative, they still have a grandmother who battled breast cancer and a mother with such a high risk that she opted to have a prophylactic mastectomy," she says. "I want them to always remind their doctors of that family history."

The key is to always be open with your children and make sure they know they can turn to you for help when it comes to their cancer risk. But eventually, as with everything in life, you'll have to let go. All you can do is give your children the resources and information they need and hope that they'll make the best choices for themselves (even if you'd prefer that they make a different choice).

One last note: If and when your child does get tested, it's important that you seek help with handling the results, too. At that point, you might be inclined not to deal with your own remorse, fear, and other emotions because you're so focused on helping your son or daughter deal with his or hers. Talk to a genetic counselor or therapist separately to help you cope with the news.

guilt factor

When a woman (or a man, for that matter) tests positive for a BRCA gene mutation, it takes on a whole different meaning when she (or he) has children. Not only are parents worried about their own mortality, but they have the added pressure of knowing they may have passed the same fate on to their children. "People often feel tremendous guilt over passing on an altered gene to their child, even though they understand they had no control over the matter," explains Beth Peshkin, a genetic counselor at Georgetown University's Lombardi

Comprehensive Cancer Center in Washington, D.C. Amy, for example, says, "I'm very worried that I might have passed the gene on to my children, especially my daughter. She's starting to develop, and deep down I'm petrified about what she might go through. I'd feel so guilty if she had to deal with all the issues I had to face. But I don't want to admit it. I'd hate for my mom to feel that way about me."

Lisa understands that point of view all too well. "After my mother tested positive for BRCA2, we both just assumed I had the mutation, too," she says. "So when our genetics expert told us that I was negative, we were both in shock. And then my mother started weeping. She hugged me tight and whispered, 'The best gift I ever gave you was not giving you that gene.' The thought that she might have passed it on to me—and possibly my children—was just eating away at her. Of course, I wouldn't want my mother to feel that kind of guilt. I know it's out of her hands. But I also know that if I had tested positive, I would have felt the same way about possibly passing the gene on to my children."

For that reason, Suzanne feels blessed that she won't transmit the BRCA mutation to her daughter, Nina, who is adopted. "Years ago, when I was dealing with infertility and going through in vitro fertilization, I was devastated," says Suzanne. "I couldn't understand why this was happening to me. But then, when I found out I had tested positive, one of my first thoughts was: 'Thank God I don't have to be concerned that I passed this on to Nina.' That's an enormous weight that I don't have to face like Amy and Rori do."

Not only do moms blame themselves for having passed on the gene. They also feel culpable that they've "opened Pandora's box" by getting tested, because that means that now their children have to deal with the consequences—often at a much younger age than they themselves had to. For instance, a woman who tests positive at forty-five might already be married and done having children. But if she has a twenty-year-old daughter, that daughter might then feel pressure to get tested.

And if she's positive, too, she might feel rushed to get married and have a baby so she could subsequently have her ovaries removed. In other words, women believe it's their fault that the inherited mutation might influence many more of their sons' and daughters' life decisions than it did their own.

Another common reason moms feel guilty, regardless if they're BRCA-positive or -negative, is that they have to "take a leave of absence" from their lives when having a prophylactic surgery, as Lisa puts it. Even if a woman is in the hospital for a day or two for an oophorectomy or mastectomy, recovery can take weeks. Lisa, Mayde, Amy, Rori, and Suzanne all traveled from Florida to New York for their mastectomies, and they agree that being away from their kids was one of the most difficult aspects of the whole ordeal. "When I told my kids I had to go away for a week, they seemed more upset about that than my surgery itself," says Lisa, who, at the time, had never spent more than a night away from her children. "I felt awful and did what I could to make them feel comfortable while I was gone. But even when I returned home and was healing, I still felt helpless that I couldn't immediately be my old self. After being gone for what wound up being two weeks because I had complications, all my kids wanted to do was kiss me and hug me, but I had to tell them they couldn't sit on my lap. I wasn't supposed to lift my arms, so if they said they wanted cereal and milk for breakfast, I had to tell them to get it themselves. I was so upset and incredibly frustrated."

It's important to note that not every parent sees a high risk for breast or ovarian cancer as her cross to bear. Rori says that she'd feel sick if she passed the genetic mutation on to any of her three kids, but she refuses to feel guilty about it. "I can't blame myself for something I can't control," she says. "If anything, I feel like I'll be in a good place to make it easier for my children if they are, in fact, positive because I've been through it all before."

Men and guilt: Women aren't the only people struggling with guilt. Dads and grandfathers who pass their altered BRCA gene on to their daughters and granddaughters can blame themselves just as much as, if not more than, women do, says Larsen Haidle. "Sometimes it's harder on men because they feel like they get by lucky," she explains. "Their cancer risks are nowhere near what their daughters' risks would be by having the mutation. And they don't have to weigh options like preventative surgery and chemoprevention." Also, when a mom passes a genetic mutation on to her daughter, she can offer support and advice on what to do because, as Rori says, she's already gone down that path. But men often feel isolated because they just can't relate to what their daughter is going through.

talking to your kids about surgery

If you choose to have a prophylactic surgery, it can be very difficult figuring out how to explain your decision to your children. A lot of what you say depends on their ages and maturity level. No one knows your kids as well as you do, so tell them whatever you think they can handle, which is usually enough to explain what's going on without overwhelming or confusing them. For instance, when telling her preschooler, Emmy, about her mastectomy, Lisa spoke in very simple terms. "I told her that I was going to the hospital to make sure that what happened to Grandma didn't happen to me, too," Lisa says. "I also explained that I wasn't sick, but that when I got home I might seem a little tired and that she couldn't pull on me. She seemed okay with that." Suzanne told her daughter, Nina, who was seven at the time, the same thing. During such discussions with your children, you might want to acknowledge that your having surgery might seem frightening. But then reassure them that you're having the operation only because you are trying to stay healthy.

However, older children often need a more elaborate explanation. Mayde remembers that when trying to figure out how to reduce her risk, she was very emotional and constantly on the computer researching her options. Her daughter, Phoebe, who was then nine years old, realized that something was up. "Phoebe's friend had just lost her mother to colon cancer, so Phoebe was very aware of what this disease can do," Mayde recalls. "She came over to me one day, put her hand on mine, looked me in the eyes, and nervously said, 'Tell me the truth. Do you have breast cancer?'

"'Absolutely not,' I said. 'I have to prevent cancer, but I don't have it.'

"'Are you sure?' Phoebe asked.

"'I have never lied to you,' I said. 'I am very sure that I do not have breast cancer, but I do have some cells in me that can turn cancerous, so I'm removing them.'

"'What do you have to do?' she asked.

"'I have to have the inside of my breasts scooped out and then have fake ones put in,' I explained.

"Phoebe said, 'Implants? Oh, that's no big deal. I just read that Lindsay Lohan got those.'"

Mayde's story is just one example. Below are some general tips on broaching the subject of surgery with your children. (Of course, a genetic counselor can help facilitate such discussions between you and any member of your family.)

Keep it simple, but don't conceal the truth: Sometimes older children will ask direct questions, particularly about how

they're going to be affected. If they think you're not answering them honestly, they might become more fearful. Amy says
that at the time of her surgery, her kids were younger, so
she just sat them down and told them she was having an
operation so she wouldn't get sick. However, now that her
daughter, Marley, is twelve, she's starting to ask Amy about
her mastectomy. "She'll say, 'Will I have breast cancer? Will I
need this surgery?'" says Amy. "It breaks my heart, but I tell
her honestly, 'I hope not.'" Lisa's daughter Gabby also asks if
she'll ever need to have a mastectomy. "I'll never say never, but
I tell her it's highly unlikely and nothing she needs to worry
about now," Lisa says.

Talk to your kids when *they're* ready. You might plan a discussion with them and they'll have no interest at the time, but
then they'll hear about breast cancer on the news or in school
and they'll start asking questions. In other words, you have
to be prepared for spontaneous conversations. For instance,
Mayde says her son, Morley, was very nonchalant when she
told him about her surgery. His response was a blasé "Oh,
okay," she says. And after her operation he was very clingy
to her, but he didn't really talk about it. But now, years later,
every once in a while they'll be driving in the car and Morley,
now twelve, will want to discuss the surgery again. "When he
hears about a celebrity who was diagnosed with breast cancer,
he'll say, 'She has cancer, but you didn't. Right Mom?'" says
Mayde. "And I take the time to reassure him once again."

Encourage them to open up. If you find your kids aren't asking
any questions at all, adds Beth Peshkin, it may be important
to gently help them to articulate their fears and concerns. "You
might want to ask them questions like 'What do you think
this means for you?' and draw out some of those feelings," she
says. "If they have seen Grandma die from breast cancer and

Mom having a mastectomy, a teen may feel very fatalistic and think it's a foregone conclusion that this will happen to her, too. You want to avoid her holding all of that in."

Don't forget about body image. As a girl reaches puberty and starts developing, it can be especially difficult for her to adjust to her changing body if other women in the family were diagnosed with breast cancer (particularly at a young age). That's why it's important to explain that breasts are nothing to be ashamed of. Amy says she needs to have such a conversation with her daughter. "I think Marley is scared about developing breasts because they are a constant reminder of the possibility of breast cancer," Amy says. "I know I need to reassure her as soon as possible. I just haven't found the time to have such a profound discussion."

Stay positive. Sometimes it's not *what* you tell your children, but *how* you tell them that has the greatest bearing on their reactions. "When I told my kids about my oophorectomy, I didn't want them to be afraid, especially since they knew their grandmother had died of ovarian cancer and their aunt had battled it," says Rori. "I sat them down separately and said, 'Mommy is going in for surgery, but it's not something I have to do. It's something I'm choosing to do to stay healthy, and I feel good about my decision.' I kept repeating, 'I am not sick,' and I gave them the same speech the following year when I had my mastectomy. I think the way I presented the information made it an easier pill for them to swallow."

a lesson in empowerment

While finding out you have a high risk for breast cancer can be earth-shattering, not all women view the news as a glass half-empty. And that's the message many moms want to convey to their children. "I don't necessarily see having the mutation as something we need to fear," says Rori. "It's not a death sentence, but knowing about it does make you more informed and likely to take care of your health. I'm just so thankful that we have this knowledge—it's a gift that those before us did not have. If my mother had known she was at risk, she would have likely had her ovaries removed and she'd still be alive. So if my kids have inherited my risk, too, I'll try to turn it into something positive and teach them what they can do with that information."

Previvors often see their actions, whether it's healthy living, surveillance, chemoprevention, or surgery, as a powerful lesson for their kids. "I don't think my daughter, Nina, really understands what I did," says Suzanne, referring to her prophylactic mastectomy. "But someday I think she'll realize you can't always sit back and wait for doctors to direct your health care. You have to grab the bull by its horns and do whatever you have to do to protect yourself. My mother was a tough woman who wasn't afraid of anything, and people always tell me I inherited her strength and guts. I'd like to think that, by having my surgery, I'm showing my daughter that I'm carrying on that tradition of strong women in my family."

For Mayde, she wanted to prove to her kids that the surgery she had was nothing like the horrific mastectomy her mother, Blossom, had gone through decades earlier. "When I returned home from the hospital, the kids came running to the door and collapsed in my arms," Mayde recalls. "They had been so concerned, and it felt like a triumphant moment when they saw that I was completely fine. I think they were proud of me."

Lisa sees her journey as a way to raise awareness among her kids. "I always drill it into them to eat well, exercise, and live a healthy lifestyle," she says. "And, even though she's only thirteen, I've started teaching Gabby that when she's older she has to take charge of her health. Also, I've been taking her to the Susan G. Komen Race for the Cure every year—in part to honor my mother, but also to make sure she feels like she's part of the cause." Amy adds that her daughter already seems to understand the importance of such support. "Marley points out when someone is wearing a pink ribbon, and she always wants to buy necklaces, bracelets, or anything that benefits breast cancer charities," Amy says. "She even has a pink Kooky pen that has a ribbon on it."

There are plenty of other ways to help your kids feel empowered themselves, particularly by giving them little chores or projects to do so they don't feel uninvolved. For instance, while you're recovering after a surgery, your children can clean up their rooms and assist with cooking dinner. Mayde says her son, Morley, and daughter, Phoebe, made a scrapbook of pictures they took of themselves while she was away so she wouldn't feel like she missed out on anything. And Lisa says her two older kids, Ben and Gabby, were her "little helpers," opening the refrigerator for her, geting dishes out of the cabinet, and even taking care of their little sister, Emmy.

Ultimately, Rori says she feels most empowered by not letting the issues she has dealt with overshadow the rest of her life. "Some people say our high risk for breast cancer (and, in my case, ovarian cancer) and the way we tackle that risk is a legacy we leave to our children," Rori says. "I don't agree. When I think of my mother, I don't focus on genetics or her battles with cancer. Instead, I look at how she lived her life, with such zest, passion, and bravery. To me, that's her legacy. And that's the kind of legacy I want to leave to my sons and my daughter."

a promising future

Just a few decades ago, there were no proven interventions for breast cancer chemoprevention, surveillance rates were painfully poor, and a mastectomy typically meant mutilation. Meanwhile, assessing a woman's risk of breast cancer was somewhat of a shot in the dark. It's amazing how far we've come in a short time, and we can only imagine what options will be available to future generations. (Even talk of a vaccine isn't that far-fetched anymore.)

The truth is, many innovative tools are on the way, and some are already here. In most cases, it's a matter of waiting to see which ones pan out. But it's also worth asking your doctor which newer techniques might be available to you. One of the best ways to take advantage of promising options is by getting involved with clinical trials, which are research studies that test the efficacy and safety of new drugs, surgical procedures, tests, and other means of screening for or preventing cancer. "Only a fraction of the women who could be involved in clinical trials choose to do so," says Eric Winer, M.D., chief scientific advisor for Susan G. Komen for the Cure, and director of the breast oncology center at Dana-Farber Cancer Institute in Boston. "But if you're comfortable participating in one, you can help move the field of breast cancer prevention forward while potentially getting the best medical care." You can find out which clinical trials are currently available at www.clinicaltrials.gov.

Experts agree that when it comes to determining breast cancer risk as well as improving surveillance and risk-reducing measures, it's an evolution not a revolution. Here's a look at what options might be available to previvors down the road:

great strides in genetics

When it comes to the world of genetics, this is just the beginning. Researchers have been continually finding new genes that may help determine who is at risk for everything from blindness and brain aneurisms to stomach cancer, Alzheimer's disease, and diabetes. Each finding carries its own issues, its own set of dilemmas among patients, and its own promises for great advancements in how these diseases are detected, treated, and possibly prevented. Here's how this explosion of knowledge might specifically affect breast cancer:

BETTER ACCURACY

Though rare, no other genetic mutations have been found that will confer as much risk for breast cancer as BRCA1 and BRCA2 (which are considered major predisposition genes). And most experts don't believe they will. What they do think they'll find are other areas in our DNA that are more common and affect risk, though to a much lesser degree. For instance, some genes don't necessarily affect a woman's risk of breast cancer by themselves, but they *can* when a woman also has a BRCA mutation. These modifier genes could explain why some women with such hereditary risk get breast cancer, some get ovarian cancer, some get both, and others don't get cancer at all. It's the combination of genes that's key. "Right now, we tell a woman with a BRCA mutation that she has '*up to* an 87 percent chance of getting breast cancer,' but we don't know if she actually has 87 percent odds, or 30 percent odds, or somewhere in between," says Angela Trepanier, past president of the National Society of Genetic Counselors. "With modifiers, we may be able to be much more specific. For instance, we might be able to tell a woman she has a 56 percent chance of getting breast cancer, so when she's weighing whether to do surgery, surveillance, or chemoprevention, that information can help her make a better informed decision."

You also might start hearing about single nucleotide polymorphisms (SNPs). SNPs are DNA sequence variations that can occur within genes or in other areas of the genome. Though most SNPs don't cause any discernable differences between people, some may be responsible for distinctions such as our eye or hair color. Scientists have also begun to identify SNPs that may be associated with an increased chance of developing certain diseases, like breast cancer. In terms of breast cancer, this newer class of discoveries confers only a slight increase in risk— very different from BRCA mutations—but they're much more common. Essentially, it's thought that SNPs can serve as markers because they're often near genes associated with particular diseases. Eventually, these SNPs will be linked to the genes they modify, which will allow researchers to better calculate their effect on an individual's risk and target therapies, explains Kenneth Offit, M.D., chief of clinical genetics service at Memorial Sloan-Kettering Cancer Center in New York City.

Experts have already found several genetic modifiers, and they predict that in the next few years, they'll find up to one hundred in total that can affect a woman's odds of getting breast cancer. In fact, Rebecca Sutphen, M.D., recent director of clinical genetics at Moffitt Cancer Center in Tampa, estimates that up to 50 percent of all breast cancer cases will have at least some genetic link. The hope is that someday we'll be able to test for a panel of genes related to breast cancer that can more accurately determine our risk.

PERSONALIZED MEDICINE

Researchers expect that in the next decade or so we'll all have access to full-genome sequencing, meaning that genetics experts will be able to read every letter of our DNA and know as much as they can about our genetic makeup. This groundbreaking development will allow individuals to find out if they're at risk not only for breast cancer but for a whole host of other diseases. Sequencing will likely give us information about relatively common genes and SNPs that raise a woman's chances of getting breast cancer (though to a much lesser degree than BRCA).

And once that happens, we'll be that much closer to personalized medicine, which is essentially using a person's genetic profile to provide the right treatment or screening at the right time. "The idea is that we will have targeted approaches for the prevention of breast cancer based on genes we're discovering now and those we will in the future," explains Dr. Offit. "For instance, researchers might be able to develop drugs based on whichever genes you have that are altered and cause risk for diseases."

GREATER AWARENESS

One of the main goals of the genetics field, as well as this book for that matter, is awareness. And experts say that that's key when it comes to preventing breast cancer or catching it as early as possible. "A lot of times, a woman might have a strong family history and a high risk for breast cancer, but it comes to her attention only when she herself gets breast cancer," says Angela Trepanier. "We want to avoid that happening and identify people *before* they get diagnosed. And as we discover more genes and eventually have full-genome sequencing, almost everyone will be able to know their risk statistics earlier in life."

Take people with BRCA mutations, for instance. Though between one in three hundred and one in eight hundred people have these mutations, less than 5 percent of those carriers are aware that they do, says Dr. Sutphen. For that reason, some experts believe that genetic testing should be conducted on a much larger scale. "Our goal should be to find all people who are BRCA carriers so we can prevent cancer [or catch it early] among that population," says Steven Narod, M.D., one of the leading BRCA researchers in the world and director of the Familial Breast Cancer Research Unit at Women's College Research Institute in Toronto. "My idea of success is that everyone with a mutation has the opportunity to be tested. For instance, we need to identify the relatives of people who already know they have it."

Many nonprofit organizations and advocates aim to help raise awareness among women at risk. And in 2009, the American College of Obstetricians and Gynecologists and the Society of Gynecologic Oncologists began recommending that their members routinely assess their patient's odds of breast and ovarian cancer to help determine who might need further risk assessment. "This awareness will hopefully lead to better services and ultimately more targeted therapies that go beyond surgical prevention," says Trepanier. "I think we've only scratched the surface right now."

A TRICKY ROAD

While this profusion of knowledge about genetics is exciting, now the challenge is how we translate it into medical care. "We need to share this information with people without frightening them," says Angela Bradbury, M.D., director of the Margaret Dyson Family Risk Assessment Program at Fox Chase Cancer Center in Philadelphia. "The key is to make sure high-risk people adopt behaviors to protect themselves, but we don't want healthy people living like they have a disease. We hope this research in the field of genetics will help doctors advise patients and their families."

One part of that equation is the arrival of direct-to-consumer tests that look at SNPs, as described earlier in this chapter. For instance, for several hundred dollars, companies called deCODEme and 23andMe can tell you for which diseases you might be at risk. However, the question remains how valuable this information might be. Some experts think this information will shape the future of medicine. Others say the tests have no place if their findings won't change a person's medical management. "I'm all for people taking control of their health care, but we don't yet know if this information is a good estimate of a woman's risk," says Angela Trepanier. "The problem with SNP testing is that we don't have all the pieces of the puzzle. For instance, what if the SNPs we currently know about show that a woman has a higher risk for breast cancer, and that person becomes highly anxious based on that information? But who's to say that in a few years we won't find more SNPs linked with breast cancer that actually lower that woman's risk of the disease. It's hard to make medical recommendations based on these uncertainties."

The world of genetics isn't without other controversies either. For instance, there has been considerable debate about whether or not a company, namely Myriad, can and should own patents on genes such as BRCA1 and BRCA2. While Myriad is the only entity that can test for these genetic mutations, some argue that such a monopoly prohibits other companies from creating less expensive BRCA tests. Also, because there's only one test, patients can't get a second opinion before making decisions about how to deal with their risk. In 2009, this debate came to a head when the American Civil Liberties Union and the Public Patent Foundation initiated a lawsuit against Myriad charging that the BRCA patents are invalid. Then, in 2010, a federal court ruled that indeed they are. However, the case will likely be appealed, and it might be years before a final decision is reached in court. As genetics becomes more complicated, more issues such as this will likely arise.

Bottom line: Genetics is an ever-changing field, and its future promises to be an exhilarating one. However, you shouldn't try to navigate these waters without the help of an expert. "What we've discovered so far is just a prelude to what will be a far more complex period of interpretation," says Dr. Offit. "Individuals will require the expertise of health care professionals to decipher the meaning of this avalanche of genomic information."

LIFESTYLE CHANGES

The jury is still out regarding how much of your breast cancer risk is genetic and how much is affected by your environment (which can range from lifestyle choices such as what you eat and how much you exercise to your exposure to estrogen, radiation, and even sunlight). However, researchers are continually trying to find an answer. For instance, a study of twins in Scandinavia found that about 70 percent of breast cancers are influenced by environmental factors. A recent Canadian study found that among women with BRCA mutations, eating a diversity of fruits and vegetables might be associated with a decreased risk of breast cancer. And the University of Pennsylvania is doing research to determine the effects exercise can have on breast cancer risk among young women who have elevated odds of getting the disease. However, there have been no definitive studies that can pinpoint exactly which environmental elements affect which particular people, says Rachel Ballard-Barbash, M.D., associate director of the National Cancer Institute's applied research program and an expert on the link between diet, weight, exercise, and cancer. The good news is that we're starting to learn more about the relationship between a person's genes and environmental factors. "While it is very clear that genes are important to cancer, the genes must be expressed, which means they must produce proteins that influence a cell's growth and function to influence health," explains Dr. Ballard-Barbash. "Increasingly, research is demonstrating that our environmental exposures, including health habits, have a critical role in determining if genes are expressed. We now understand that it is not only the presence of genes but whether or not they are expressed that influences disease, including breast cancer."

The theory is that when we have a better understanding of which genetic factors are highly predictive of a person developing breast cancer, we will be better able to determine which lifestyle factors can affect that risk. And at that point, the medical community can make concrete recommendations for those particular high-risk women. For now, experts suggest that all women (and men, for that matter) maintain a healthy weight, exercise, eat a balanced diet, and limit alcohol to ward off a multitude of illnesses. "We can't say with absolute accuracy which diseases a person is going to get," says Dr. Ballard-Barbash. "So the trick is to practice habits that will improve your overall health and possibly be beneficial against many different diseases."

breast cancer screening: on the horizon

When breast cancer is caught early, the survival rate is higher than 95 percent. So, naturally, the goal is to try to diagnose this disease as soon as possible. While mammograms remain the staple of breast cancer screening, experts are always searching for technology that can better detect tumors (especially among women with dense breasts). In 2007, the American Cancer Society started recommending MRI (magnetic resonance imaging) in addition to mammograms for women who have a breast cancer risk higher than 20 percent. Currently, MRI is still the best bet for women who need that extra screening, yet this test can run thousands of dollars and can be contraindicated for those with a pacemaker or renal (kidney) disease. A conventional MRI can also be very uncomfortable for women who are claustrophobic (though some machines now have a more open design). The good news is that there is a whole slew of other breast cancer screening tools in the works that can also supplement (or improve the accuracy of) regular mammograms. Some look promising; others don't. And overall, more work needs to be done to determine such factors as accurate false-positive and false-negative rates. Techniques to watch for include:

MOLECULAR BREAST IMAGING

Mammograms and ultrasound study the architecture or anatomical structure of breasts, but this new shift in breast cancer screening looks at breast tissue on a cellular level. The idea behind molecular breast imaging is that often by the time a tumor has grown large enough to be detectable on an X-ray, it might not be useful for patients with more aggressive forms of breast cancer, says Barbara Galen, a program director of the Cancer Imaging Program at the NCI. Molecular breast imaging uses contrast agents to show cancerous tissue, which is more metabolically active than normal tissue. Here are two major developments in this area:

- **Breast-specific gamma imaging (BSGI).** With this technique, a radiologist will inject into a woman's bloodstream a small amount of radioactive tracer, which is then absorbed by cells in the body. A gamma camera then tracks cancerous cells, which, because of their high metabolism, will take up more of the tracer than will healthy cells, making them more conspicuous. BSGI is considerably less inexpensive than MRI, and it can pick up lesions as small as one millimeter. Some studies have found it highly sensitive at detecting cancer; one study showed it more sensitive than mammogram and MRI at detecting DCIS (ductal carcinoma in situ), while another found it more sensitive than mammogram, MRI, and ultrasound at detecting a breast cancer that starts in the milk-producing glands and spreads (invasive lobular carcinoma).

BSGI also appears to have a greater specificity than MRI. It can be more comfortable than a mammogram, as it typically involves mild compression, but the whole process takes thirty minutes to one hour. Experts say that the only side effect is the slight exposure to radiation.

- **Positron emission mammography (PEM).** This technology works similarly to BSGI in that it analyzes the metabolic activity in breasts. With PEM, a technician injects a patient with a radioactive glucose sugar, which is used by cells for energy. Cancer cells absorb more of the sugar than healthy cells do and, in turn, they're highlighted on the PEM image. In one study of patients with breast cancer, this method successfully detected malignancies in 100 percent of fatty breasts, 93 percent of dense breasts, 85 percent of extremely dense breasts, 90 percent of premenopausal women, 94 percent of postmenopausal women, and 93 percent of women regardless of whether or not they ever took hormone replacement therapy. As with BSGI, PEM can involve less compression than a traditional mammogram, though it, too, may take longer and involves exposure to radiation.

3-D MAMMOGRAMS (TOMOSYNTHESIS)

This technology aims to improve the accuracy of mammograms. Whereas a traditional mammogram is a two-dimensional image, this digital technique involves an X-ray tube that moves around the breasts in an arc and takes pictures of each breast in multiple one-millimeter layers. Those images are then combined into a three-dimensional series. One of the advantages of tomosynthesis is that it can avoid tissue overlap, which occurs with traditional mammograms. It's like looking at a loaf of bread in slices rather than the whole loaf at once. If there's a raisin in the middle of the loaf, you're more likely to see it if you look at it in slices. Another benefit of this technology is that it can detect very small cancers, particularly in women with dense breasts. Researchers are also examining whether tomosynthesis can possibly involve reduced breast compression, making it less painful for women than traditional mammography. Tomosynthesis has a radiation exposure similar to that of regular digital mammograms, which is slightly less than that of the two molecular breast imaging techniques mentioned above, says Kathryn Evers, M.D., director of breast imaging at Fox Chase Cancer Center in Philadelphia.

AND FURTHER DOWN THE ROAD . . .

We're not going to wake up tomorrow and women won't need mammograms anymore. But at some point, we'll have something as simple as a blood test that can tell if a woman has breast cancer, says Dr. Evers. There's talk of optical scanning (whereby a doctor could use handheld probes or fluorescent lights to know where a tumor is located), as well as a process that examines blood vessels in tumors. Also, based on a patient's risk factors, doctors may continue to make more personal recommendations for screening. For instance, someone with an extremely low risk might need a mammogram only every few years, while someone with a BRCA mutation might need a few tests biannually. "Cancer screening is not a one-size-fits-all," explains Dr. Galen of the NCI. "We'll have to examine all the technology available in our arsenal in different combinations to figure out what is right for each person."

advances in chemoprevention

So far, raloxifene and tamoxifen are the only drugs approved for reducing breast cancer risk. There are other agents being investigated, such as anti-inflammatory drugs, statins (cholesterol-lowering drugs), and vitamin A derivatives that might have the potential to impact the development of breast cancer, says Therese Bevers, M.D., medical director of the Cancer Prevention Center at M. D. Anderson Cancer Center in Houston. However, those are way down the pipeline, as much more research needs to be done.

The only drugs even close to FDA approval for breast cancer prevention are aromatase inhibitors, which are currently used to help prevent breast cancer recurrences in postmenopausal women who have already had the disease. Here's how they work: Aromatase is an enzyme the body needs to produce estrogen. These aromatase inhibitors block this enzyme, and, consequentially, the production of estrogen. So far, they show promise in being better at preventing breast cancer than tamoxifen or raloxifene, with fewer side effects, says Dr. Bevers, but until all of the possible risks and benefits are known, doctors have to prescribe one of the two FDA-approved drugs they know works.

What's the next step? Some experts say that raising awareness of tamoxifen among premenopausal women is key, particularly since few women are taking advantage of the option. For those with BRCA1, that's understandable, as the drug doesn't appear to lower risk in women with the genetic mutation. However, for BRCA2-positive women or those without a known mutation but with other risk factors, tamoxifen is a great choice, says Leslie Ford, M.D., a researcher in the NCI's Division of Cancer Prevention who led the initial study of the drug. "Tamoxifen is a missed opportunity for young women," she says. "Taking it for five years can offer considerable protection against breast cancer." And while women are wary of the agent because of certain side effects, such as uterine cancer, deep vein thrombosis, and pulmonary embolism, the truth is those symptoms are primarily seen in women older than fifty. In other words, premenopausal women have the benefits of tamoxifen without any major risks. Bottom line:

There needs to be more education for women and physicians that chemoprevention is a viable option for high-risk women.

AND FURTHER DOWN THE ROAD . . .

"As researchers, we hope to eventually find a drug with the highest breast cancer risk reduction with the fewest side effects—that would be the Holy Grail," says Dr. Bevers. "Until then, it's a tradeoff. We have to find acceptable balances between risks and benefits." The hope is that someday a field called pharmacogenomics will be able to tailor treatment to each person differently. "Once we have a better understanding of how genes work, we can have therapies targeted specifically for each genetic mutation," explains Angela Trepanier, past president of the National Society of Genetic Counselors. "For instance, if we understand what protein or molecule is missing, we can try to replace it without any side effects. Designing medication based on a person's genetic makeup will happen, but it's a long way off." Early studies of a class of drugs called Parp inhibitors have shown it to work particularly well among women with BRCA mutations who already have breast cancer. Once they're proven to work for the treatment of breast cancer, maybe the next step will be for researchers to study their role in breast cancer prevention.

new strides in prophylactic mastectomies

When it comes to prophylactic mastectomies, there are already techniques available that can change the face of this field (as discussed in Chapter 6). In some cases, it's a matter of them becoming more available; in others, it's a question of validating the research that has already been done. But overall, experts say more women are considering prophylactic mastectomies because an increasing number of surgeons are focusing on the aesthetic beauty of the outcome. Instead of simply providing a mound that can fill a bra, these new techniques help doctors create breasts that are natural-looking and attractive.

The goal is to take such surgical advancements and maximize their potential. "We have a long way to go even with the science that is in hand right now, as we need to continually improve success rates, cosmetic outcome, and availability," says Frank DellaCroce, M.D., co-director of the Center for Restorative Breast Surgery in New Orleans. The idea is that once the public becomes more aware of these options, they'll create a demand that, in turn, will increase commitment from surgeons across the country to respond to it. And with hope, the third hurdle—persuading insurers to compensate for these newer procedures—will come in time.

Of course, in regards to prophylactic mastectomies, removing as much breast tissue as possible is most important. However, here are some techniques that are allowing surgeons to also achieve the best cosmetic outcome:

NIPPLE SPARING

Years ago, doctors performing a mastectomy typically removed all the skin and tissue on the chest wall. However, after researchers determined that skin-sparing mastectomies were safe, they became more of a universal standard. Experts predict the same thing will likely happen with nipple-sparing procedures, in which a surgeon removes all the tissue behind the nipple and leaves only the skin behind. So far, experts have found that saving the nipple doesn't seem to lead to more breast cancer diagnoses, but more research needs to be done. "As we continue to accumulate data on the safety of this procedure, in a few years it will be as common as skin sparing," predicts Patrick Borgen, M.D., director of the Brooklyn Breast Cancer Program at Maimonides Medical Center in New York.

MICROSURGICAL PROCEDURES

As recently as ten years ago, having a flap surgery meant you had to have longer than a ten-hour operation, at least a week-long hospital stay, and possibly blood transfusions, while a good chunk of muscle was taken along with the tissue. However, with microsurgical techniques, doctors can collect fat but "dance delicately" in the area from where they remove it, says Dr. Frank DellaCroce. This procedure, during which a doctor removes tissue from one part of the body and reconnects it in the breast area, leads to less time in the hospital and a speedier recovery. While microsurgical procedures do currently exist, many doctors still have not yet learned them, which means they're not readily available to all women. "Changes in plastic surgery can be like turning a battleship," says Dr. DellaCroce. "We have new techniques, but they require a big commitment from plastic surgeons to learn and master them." In other words, more women will have access to microsurgical flap surgeries, but it might take some time.

IMPLANTS

Most women who get implants after a mastectomy have to go through the lengthy process of having expanders. As it turns out Lisa, Mayde, Amy, Rori, and Suzanne chose a rather cutting-edge procedure when they decided to have a direct-to-implant reconstruction. In such cases, the surgeon uses an acellular skin graft called AlloDerm (derived from human skin) or Strattice (derived from pig skin), to allow for immediate reconstruction (see Chapter 6 for more information). Again, says their surgeon Andrew Salzberg, M.D., who pioneered this technique, it's a matter of more physicians being willing to learn how to perform these surgeries. "A few years ago, no one was using this technique, and now I'd estimate about 20 percent of doctors are," he says. "Possibly many more will be using it in the future."

Implants themselves aren't going to change drastically, adds Dr. Salzberg, though researchers are toying with the cohesiveness of silicone implants. New products called "gummy-bear implants" are under investigation and an option for women who participate in clinical trials for the product. These implants are very firm—if you cut one in half, it would retain its shape just like a gummy bear—and some experts say they might be longer-lasting than other implants. Though available in Europe, it remains to be seen if gummy-bear implants will make it to the general market in the United States.

AND FURTHER DOWN THE ROAD . . .

Hopefully, prophylactic mastectomies someday will be a thing of the past. "While advancements in technology will allow doctors to soften the blow to patients having this surgery, that's not our goal," says Dr. Borgen. "Our goal is to eliminate the need for prophylactic mastectomies altogether by finding smarter ways to prevent this dreadful disease."

Until then, experts continually work on finding new techniques. There's one, for instance, where a surgeon could essentially suck the fat out of one area of your body and re-inject it back into your breast. In fact, the BRAVA Breast Enhancement and Shaping System is a suction device that expands the breast pocket for such a procedure without having to have surgery. However, many more tests need to be done to determine if it's safe and effective for prophylactic mastectomies. Additionally, there's talk about endoscopic mastectomies, a procedure done in Asia that allows a surgeon to perform the entire surgery through a small incision under the arm. And there's also the idea that many years from now we'll be able to create entire organs out of thin air using stem cells. Right now, some experts say this is the stuff of science fiction. But while we might not see these advancements in our lifetime, who knows what's in store for future generations?

slow but steady progress against ovarian cancer

Ovarian cancer is a tough nut to crack. It's very aggressive and spreads much faster than other diseases like breast cancer. In most cases, by the time a doctor detects a mass on the ovaries, the cancer has already spread and the patient's prognosis is poor.

When it comes to risk reduction, an oophorectomy is still the best option, though it causes a woman to lose her fertility and hormones. While there are some advancements in terms of how to perform the surgery, there are no major breakthroughs on the horizon, says David Fishman, M.D., director of the National Ovarian Cancer Early Detection Program. "Most oophorectomies today are minimally invasive, so whether done robotically or with one incision or three, the outcome is relatively the same," he says. Meanwhile, as far as chemoprevention is concerned, birth control pills are still the most effective medication used to prevent ovarian cancer, with a 50 percent or higher reduction after five or more years of lifetime use. (Again, it's not yet entirely clear whether or not those statistics apply to women with BRCA mutations.)

However, while surveillance of ovarian cancer has been notoriously difficult, there is ongoing research that hopefully will find better tools to catch ovarian cancer at stages when it's most treatable. "Screening ultrasound is by far the best tool we have to visualize the ovaries, but though it's outstanding at picking up advanced stages of cancer, it's not good at picking up smaller early lesions," explains Dr. Fishman. For that reason, experts are trying to identify new imaging technology as well as blood and urine tests that may detect this disease as early as possible.

One particularly exciting development is the use of contrast agents along with ultrasound, a technique often used in cardiology. There's a process called tumor angiogenesis by which a cancer creates its own blood supply in order for it to grow. Such vascular changes aren't seen by conventional ultrasound, but a contrast agent makes this feasible because it detects blood vessels by "lighting them up like Christmas tree lights," as Dr. Fishman puts it. Preliminary results show promise as researchers were able to pick up early cancers not detectable by ultrasound alone. The next step? "We're trying to validate this technique, and if we do, it will be a giant step forward in saving women's lives," says Dr. Fishman.

a previvor's future

The future looks bright for previvors. As the advancements and innovations in this chapter come to fruition, generations to come are going to view breast cancer differently, says Angela Trepanier, past president of the National Society of Genetic Counselors. "Those people won't have witnessed multiple family members suffering or dying from cancer," she says. "They'll see this as a disease they have control over."

Lindsay Avner, founder of Bright Pink, agrees. "This is such an exciting time, because we can identify a woman's risk and do something about it," she says. "I've met so many women who refuse to bury their heads in the sand and wait for cancer to strike. They are taking steps to protect themselves."

Also, as we identify additional causes of breast cancer, the number of previvors will only increase, which experts believe will force researchers to increase their focus on this community. "Research for a cancer cure is critical, but where we have the great potential to save lives with the technology and information we have *right now* is the area of risk assessment and risk management," says Sue Friedman, founder of FORCE. "We can figure out who is in the highest risk category and offei them the appropriate options." Adds Dr. Winer, chief scientific advisor for Susan G. Komen for the Cure, "As a growing number of women find out they have an elevated risk of breast cancer, that will result in more experts and researchers paying attention to them. This, in turn, will lead to more efforts to find new means of surveillance and risk-reducing options."

Strides have already been made in that direction. Susan G. Komen for the Cure has instituted Promise Grants, which give millions of dollars to institutions for breast cancer research. In the fiscal year 2009–2010, the grants focused solely on the prevention of breast cancer. And U.S. Representative Debbie Wasserman Schultz of Florida introduced legislation called the Education and Awareness Requires Learning Young Act (EARLY), which would raise awareness among young women about their risk for breast cancer and the importance of breast self-exams and getting regular checkups. The act also aims to educate doctors, many of whom often dismiss the possibility of breast cancer in young women because it's so rare. But when it does strike this age group, it's often more aggressive. "When doctors send these patients home, they're risking that they'll come back with breast cancer at a later stage, and more dire consequences," says Representative Wasserman Shultz, who recently had a prophylactic mastectomy and oophorectomy when she was diagnosed with breast cancer and discovered she had a BRCA2 mutation. She adds that she doesn't want to frighten women, but she wants them to know their potential risk and take steps to protect themselves. "There are millions of women younger than forty who go through life thinking they're invincible," she says. "However, when they become educated about their breast health and what their potential risk is, the more likely they'll catch breast cancer early if it strikes and survive," she says.

One expert recently said, "Cancer is still smarter than us." And while that statement may be true, women like Lisa, Mayde, Amy, Rori, and Suzanne are aiming to prove it wrong. They refuse to be outwitted by a disease they have seen win far too many battles. They choose empowerment over fear. Their mothers didn't have this great gift of knowledge or so many options to defy their fate. It's thrilling to think what the future will hold for our children.

afterword

As I first started writing this book, little did I know that I'd soon be part of a bond that Lisa, Mayde, Amy, Rori, and Suzanne have shared since that fateful morning at Dunkin' Donuts years ago. When I met these women, I learned that people like them desperately wanted, or rather needed, a book about living with a high risk for breast cancer. They explained that they wished to share their stories because they knew nothing compares with hearing that firsthand account, that raw honesty you can get only from talking to others who have been in your shoes. Their mission was to help create a book that would guide previvors through their journeys.

Over time, these brave women told me about their personal experiences. They spoke of the utter fear they felt with every mammogram, every biopsy. They wept as they walked me through their mothers' battles with cancer and, in some cases, what it's like to live without them. They recounted how they made the excruciating decision to have all of their healthy breast tissue removed. After a while, I wasn't a journalist and they the interviewees. They were my friends telling me their most intimate stories.

While getting to know these women, I've witnessed how deeply they care about one another. They feel lucky to have found one another, and now I feel blessed to know them. When we're together, there's always a lot of laughter, a lightheartedness and comfort shared solely among dear friends. We talk not only about the book, but also about our husbands, children, current events, and our favorite TV shows. But there's always a reminder of how we know one another. On one recent occasion, we were just settling down for lunch when Mayde's cell phone rang. It was yet another high-risk young woman Mayde had recently met who was seeking guidance; in this case, the caller wanted to know what kind of post-mastectomy bras she should buy. Within seconds, this girl was offered five different opinions. But that was just one person they were helping. With this book, we're hoping to reach out to so many others.

Lisa, Mayde, Amy, Rori, and Suzanne each said that sharing their stories for the book was cathartic, but that it was difficult and draining at times. Though they all "made it to the other side," as they put it, the experience was far from easy, and reliving it was often a struggle. But ultimately, they felt it was necessary in order to help other women just starting to confront their risk. And while they opened their hearts and spoke of the choices they made, countless researchers, doctors, and other medical professionals provided a wealth of knowledge on a topic that has only recently entered the limelight. These experts and organizations, like FORCE, Susan G. Komen for the Cure, and Bright Pink, helped start the conversation with women about their risk, raising awareness. This book hopes to continue that dialogue.

Today, these five women each say they have a new lease on life because they're no longer living with the looming threat of breast cancer (and in Rori's case, ovarian cancer) hanging over their heads. The stress and anxiety that had been such an integral part of their very existence is gone. Their breast cancer risk doesn't define them anymore, and they feel an overwhelming sense of relief.

As for their surgeries, they're grateful that they found a reconstructive option that made them feel whole again. Lisa says that it's as though her breasts were pillows, and her doctors simply replaced the stuffing. And while they each dream of a day when prophylactic mastectomies are a thing of the past, they are happy with their results and feel like they can move on.

Yet Suzanne and Amy still have another hurdle to face. They know that because of their BRCA mutations, they have a much higher than average risk for ovarian cancer. And since the medical community can't yet offer them good surveillance options, they feel forced to have their ovaries removed, just like Rori did. Amy says that because of her newfound single status, she has too much on her plate right now to even consider surgery. And Suzanne says she hasn't had the operation because she's frightened about going into premature menopause. However, both plan to take that next step, and they acknowledge that they won't feel at ease until they do.

Of course, Rori and Amy still worry about their children because they know there's a 50/50 chance each of their sons and daughters have inherited their risk. (Suzanne doesn't have that concern because her daughter is adopted.) They worry, but they also acknowledge that there's nothing they can do but someday share the knowledge they've garnered with their kids. We can only hope the options for all of our children are so much better down the road, just as the options have dramatically improved in past decades.

While working on this book, we each couldn't help but think of those who could have been helped and possibly saved if they had had the medical information we have today. And though women still fear breast cancer more than any other disease, the truth is we can turn that fear into empowerment. We can fight this terrible illness before it even strikes by knowing our risk and making informed decisions. We can take charge. That doesn't mean you have to make the same choices as the women in this book or anyone else. In fact, you don't have to do a thing. But learning this vital information for yourself, your children, or other loved ones gives you control over a disease that has been winning for way too long. These are your decisions to make, and the road you choose can be a very difficult one. But along the way, know that you're not alone.

acknowledgments

First and foremost, I owe an enormous debt of gratitude to Mayde Wiener, Rori Clark, Suzanne Citere, Amy Rosenthal, and Lisa Marton. These five inspiring women generated the idea for this book, and they gave me the tremendous honor of writing it. Their honesty, candidness, and passion are what gives *Previvors* its heart.

Mayde, thank you for spreading your knowledge about breast cancer risk to so many women who need guidance. You are truly a maven. Rori, your optimism and positive outlook are infectious; I am touched by your kindness. Suzanne, I appreciate your strength. You give your opinion with conviction, but you always do so gracefully. Amy, it wasn't easy for you to open up, and I thank you for doing so. Your sense of humor helped me get through even the toughest of chapters. And Lisa, I am grateful to you for spearheading this project. From the beginning, you put the pieces in place that took this book from an idea to a reality. You were my sounding board, and I thank you for always listening. To the five of you, thank you for your confidence in me. I am blessed to have worked with you.

Together, we have many people to thank who made *Previvors* possible. First, to Bob Shook, for being our biggest fan and guiding us from the start. To our agent, Al Zuckerman, for embracing our idea, finding it the perfect home, and taking a chance on a new author. To Maya Rock for all of your help. To Chris Fauteux for recommending me for this project. By mentioning my name to Lisa, you changed my life.

It has been such a pleasure working with Lucia Watson, our thoughtful and thorough editor. Thank you for your enthusiasm, for believing in us, and for caring so deeply about this important topic. Much appreciation to Miriam Rich for your kindness, support, and diligent work. And thank you to the rest of our brilliant team at Penguin: Bill Shinker, Megan Newman, Lisa Johnson, Lindsay Gordon, Adenike Olanrewaju, Jessica Chun, Elizabeth Wagner, and Janice Kurzius.

Dr. Kenneth Offit, thank you for writing such an eloquent and poignant foreword. Your words are the perfect introduction to the book, and we are honored that you are a part of it.

To Cheryl Runsdorf, for your incredible talent and generosity. We appreciate the time and effort you put into making our book trailer.

Sue Friedman, if it weren't for you and FORCE, the five women in this book would have never met one another. You coined the term "previvor," and you've brought the issue of hereditary breast and ovarian cancer into the limelight. You're an inspiration to us and to countless others. Lindsay Avner, through Bright Pink you've spread the message to many high-risk young women that they are not alone. Your passion and positive message are a comfort to them, and we greatly admire you for both.

All of the seventy-plus experts I interviewed for this book provided a tremendous wealth of knowledge about genetics, breast cancer risk, screening, and prevention. I am completely indebted to each of them. Some experts went over and beyond, fact-checking pages of copy, spending hours explaining intricate medical and financial details. I thank these men and women for their generous time and effort: Rebecca Sutphen, M.D., Patrick Borgen, M.D., Andrew Salzberg, M.D., Kathryn Evers, M.D., David Fishman, M.D., David Cohn, M.D., Leslie Ford, M.D., Therese Bevers, M.D., Angela Trepanier, M.S., Paul Jacobsen, Ph.D., Debbie Saslow, Ph.D., Talia Donenberg, M.S., Alvaro

Monteiro, Ph.D., Julie Margenthaler, M.D., Frank DellaCroce, M.D., Nancy Davenport-Ennis, Joy Larsen Haidle, M.S., Kathy Schilling, M.D., Jonathan Wiener, M.D., Daisy Castro, Adela Porro, R.T., and Beth Cerbone.

Also, I am grateful to the numerous medical organizations that provided up-to-the minute research, referrals, and other details for this book. I couldn't have written *Previvors* without the help of the following people: Jamie Kimbrough at the American Cancer Society; Stacy Brooks and Greg Phillips at the American College of Obstetricians and Gynecologists; Kathleen Gibson and Jeanne D'Agostino at Memorial Sloan-Kettering Cancer Center; Shawn Farley at the American College of Radiology; Kimberly Martin and Anthony Beal at the National Cancer Institute; Erin Moaratty at the Patient Advocate Foundation; Brian Hugins and Deana Dziadosz at the American Society of Plastic Surgeons; Susan Morris at the Society of Gynecologic Oncologists; Diana Quattrone at Fox Chase Cancer Center; Robbin Ray at Dana-Farber Cancer Institute; Sandi Weber at Boca Raton Community Hospital; Patty Kim at Moffitt Cancer Center; Marsha Wilson at the Gynecologic Cancer Foundation; Chris Hobson at the American Psychological Association; Jeremy Moore at the American Association for Cancer Research; Kimberly Arndt at Northwestern Memorial Hospital; Jan Testa at Ohio State University Medical Center; Eileen Widmer at the Society of Surgical Oncology; Julie Penne at the University of Texas M. D. Anderson Cancer Center; Elizabeth Goliwas Bodet at the Center for Restorative Breast Surgery. And to everyone else who helped with my research, a million thanks.

Much appreciation to Susan Rutstein for reading an early manuscript of the book and for your constant support. My infinite gratitude to my parents, Elaine and Howard Roth, for your help, guidance, and never-faltering belief in me. Thanks to my brother, Jack, for your love and encouragement, and to Debbie Klingsberg for lending me a hand. Many thanks to Anthony Jaswinski and Ann Birr for giving me the confidence that I could turn my passion for writing into a career. I couldn't have asked for a kinder, more talented mentor than Liz Brody.

acknowledgments

Thank you for your help along the way. Also, my appreciation to David France for giving me a glimpse of what it's like to be a top-notch reporter. And to Eleanor and her family, thank you for reminding me why this book is so vital.

To my biggest fans, Samantha and Zachary, thank you for your patience and your love, and for somehow understanding that my work was important even though it took precious time away from you. You both inspire me every day, and I love and cherish you more than you know.

I could never adequately thank my husband, Larry. From taking the cover and author photos and reading every draft to providing Internet support and social media guidance, you have been an integral part of this book. You've kept me grounded throughout the project, and you've always provided me with sound advice and unflinching support. I couldn't have done this without you.

The five women featured in *Previvors* wish to thank their doctors, Louise Morrell, M.D., Andrew Salzberg, M.D., Roy Ashikari, M.D., and Andrew Ashikari, M.D., and their friends and family who supported them during their surgeries and throughout the creation of this book. They would also like to thank:

LISA

Thank you to my husband, Bob, for your encouragement, understanding, love, and support. You are always there for me. To my children, Gabby, Ben, and Emmy, you mean everything to me, and I thank you for your help and for letting me work on this project. I know it took time away from you, but it was for a good cause—in memory of Grandma Arlene. Thank you, Dina, for spending so many hours listening to our stories, feeling our emotions, and eloquently capturing them on paper. Not only was it a joy spending time with you—it was also therapeutic. Thank you to my friends Liz and R. J. Shook for helping us get started with this book and for encouraging me along the way. And thanks to those who went above and beyond to contribute to *Previvors*: Chris Fauteux, Larry Port, Larry Blair, and Stephanie Robin. Great appreciation to all my dear friends and neighbors who helped me during a difficult time in my life. To Amy, thank you for inspiring my journey as a previvor and for always being a source of comfort and compassion. You, Rori, Suzanne, and Mayde mean the world to me. And to my mother, whom I miss terribly: You will always live on in my memory. I did this for you.

SUZANNE

Thank you to my guardian angels, my parents, Pat and Nina DiVasto, for sending me people who helped me along this journey—especially Mayde. To my amazing husband, Pascal, for all of his love, tenderness, and unwavering support. To my daughter, Nina, for being the reason I had the courage to do what I did (so that I'll be around to nag her for a long time!). Much appreciation to my sister, Patricia, for stepping in and helping us; Beth Cerbone for all of her hard work on my behalf; and my niece Tamara for just "getting it."

MAYDE

I thank my husband, Jonathan, who medically directed me and emotionally supported my journey to reduce my risk of breast cancer. Gratitude to my mother, Blossom, who taught me the importance of being vigilant with my breast care. To my children, Phoebe and Morley, who inspired me to take the preemptive strike and undergo prophylactic surgery. To my sister, Randi, many hugs for taking care of my family while I was recuperating. To Dr. Penny Wise Budoff, my mentor, who taught me that women should respect their ability to make difficult choices and to face their problems with bravery. To two special women I met at the beginning of my path, Debbi O'Shea and Sharon Kulik, who with their kindness and support guided me to take the right steps. I could never thank you enough.

AMY

Thank you to my grandmother Ada, whom I never met but always wished I could have; to my mother, Anne, an amazingly strong woman; and to my college roommate Randi, who is a breast cancer survivor. Grandma, Mom, and Randi, you each helped me become the person I am today. To my children, Ryan, Marley, and Dylan, you are the three main reasons I went through this journey. I am also lucky to have a supportive family: my sister and her husband, Tracey and Jay; my brother and his wife, Kenny and Nicole; and my dad, Larry, whose famous words are "Everything will work out." Dad, you were right. Thank you to Dina for working so hard, and for your patience and dedication. And thanks to Lisa, Rori, Suzanne, and Mayde, four women with whom I share a special camaraderie. All of you hold a special place in my heart.

RORI

Thank you to my husband, Terry, for your constant support and love, and to my children, Ryland, Linden, and Jensen, for giving me strength and courage. I couldn't have done this without you. Thank you to my sister Nancie for always listening. To my mother-in-law, Brenda (Meems), for guiding me and helping me. Your love means everything. Thank you to Talia Donenberg for sharing your knowledge, and to Dr. Mark Firestone for being so caring. Much appreciation to Kimmy for being there from the start, and to my friends Debra, Mary, and Renee, who also stood by me along the way. To Lisa Ross for always listening. A special thanks to my sister Lynne for being my true angel and for urging me to get tested. Thanks to Lisa, Mayde, Amy, and Suzanne for going through this journey with me, and to Dina for always helping me feel comfortable sharing my story. Last but not least, I thank my mother, Lois, whom I miss every day of my life. I wish I had had more time with you. To all, I love you from the bottom of my heart.

Together, Lisa, Mayde, Amy, Rori, Suzanne, and I all thank the previvors and survivors who have inspired us, and we remember those whom we wish this book could have helped. This book is for you, for our children, and for those who may someday call themselves previvors.

notes

CHAPTER TWO. LIVING IN FEAR

7 *In fact, one survey showed that women fear:* Society for Women's Health Research survey, conducted June 22–29, 2005.

7 *even though cardiovascular disease claims:* Cardiovascular disease claims more than 400,000 women's lives in the United States each year, according to the American Heart Association. Breast cancer claims around 40,000 lives each year, according to the American Cancer Society.

CHAPTER THREE. WHAT'S MY RISK?

25 *For instance, the average woman has a one-in-eight chance:* American Cancer Society, "Breast Cancer Facts and Figures 2009–2010," p. 11.

26 *can be as high as a staggering 87 percent:* Ford D, Easton DF, Bishop DT, Narod SA, Goldgar DE, Breast Cancer Linkage Consortium. "Risks of cancer in BRCA1-mutation carriers." *Lancet.* 1994 Mar 19;343(8899):692–695.

27 *Being a woman is the biggest risk factor:* American Cancer Society, "Detailed Guide: Breast Cancer: What are the risk factors for breast cancer?" www .cancer.org.

27 *The older a woman is:* American Cancer Society, "Detailed Guide: Breast Cancer: What are the risk factors for breast cancer?" www.cancer.org.

27 *Experts generally consider 5 percent to 10 percent:* American Cancer Society, "Breast Cancer Facts and Figures 2009–2010," p. 11. American Cancer Society, "Detailed Guide: Breast Cancer: What are the risk factors for breast cancer?" www.cancer.org.

28 *which is the case in from one in three hundred to one in eight hundred people:* American College of Obstetricians and Gynecologists, press release, March 20,

2009. www.acog.org. Author interviews with Rebecca Sutphen, M.D., 2009. Raičevič-Maravič L, Radulovič S. "Breast cancer susceptibility gene 1-BRCA1." *Archive of Oncology.* 2000;8(1):21–23.

28 *Some studies estimate up to an 87 percent lifetime risk . . . and up to a 44 percent lifetime risk:* Ford D, Easton DF, Bishop DT, Narod SA, Goldgar DE, Breast Cancer Linkage Consortium. "Risks of cancer in BRCA1-mutation carriers." *Lancet.* 1994 Mar 19;343(8899):692–695.

28 *increase a woman's risk of other cancers:* Breast Cancer Linkage Consortium. "Cancer risks in BRCA2 mutation carriers." *Journal of the National Cancer Institute.* 1999 Aug 4;91(15):1310–1316. Brose MS, Rebbeck TR, Calzone KA, Stopfer JE, Nathanson KL, Weber BL. "Cancer risk estimates for BRCA1 mutation carriers identified in a risk evaluation program." *Journal of the National Cancer Institute.* 2002 Sept 18;94(18):1365–1372.

29 *having this syndrome puts women at a 25 to 50 percent risk:* University of Texas M.D. Anderson Cancer Center, Patient Education Office, November 5, 2005. www.mdanderson.org. "Cowden Syndrome," www.cancer.net.

29 *People with this rare mutation have up to a 50 percent risk:* "Li-Fraumeni syndrome," Ohio State University Medical Center, www.medicalcenter.osu.edu. "Genetics and Cancer—Li-Fraumeni Syndrome," Brigham and Women's Hospital, www.brighamandwomens.org.

30 *A woman who has developed cancer in one breast:* American Cancer Society, "Detailed Guide: Breast Cancer: What are the risk factors for breast cancer?" www.cancer.org.

30 *Having one first-degree relative . . . with breast cancer doubles:* American Cancer Society, "Detailed Guide: Breast Cancer: What are the risk factors for breast cancer?" www.cancer.org.

30 *one recent study found that BRCA-negative women:* Metcalfe KA, Finch A, Poll A, Horsman D, Kim-Sing C, Scott J, Royer R, Sun P, Narod SA. "Breast cancer risks in women with a family history of breast or ovarian cancer who have tested negative for a BRCA1 or BRCA2 mutation." *British Journal of Cancer.* 2009 Jan 27;100(2):421–425. Pub. online 2008 Dec 16.

31 *White women have higher odds of developing breast cancer:* American Cancer Society, "Breast Cancer Facts and Figures 2009–2010," p. 4.

31 *Jewish people of Ashkenazi . . . descent have a one-in-forty chance:* American College of Obstetricians and Gynecologists, press release, March 20, 2009. www.acog.org.

31 *Abnormal Breast Biopsy Results:* American Cancer Society, "Breast Cancer Facts and Figures 2009–2010," p. 13.

31 *Women with LCIS:* Mayo Clinic, "Breast Cancer Risk Assessment." www.mayoclinic.org.

31 *Women who have had radiation therapy:* Travis LB, Hill D, Dores GM, Gospodarowicz M, van Leeuwen FE, Holowaty E, Glimelius B, Andersson M, Pukkala E, Lynch CF, Pee D, Smith SA, Van't Veer MB, Joensuu T, Storm H, Stovall M, Boice JD Jr., Gilbert E, Gail MH. "Cumulative absolute breast cancer risk for young women treated for Hodgkin Lymphoma." *Journal of the National Cancer Institute.* 2005;97:1428–1437.

32 *Breast Density:* Barlow WE, White E, Ballard-Barbash R, et al. "Prospective breast cancer risk prediction model for women undergoing screening mammography." *Journal of the National Cancer Institute.* 2006;98:1204–1214. American Cancer Society, "Breast Cancer Facts and Figures 2009–2010," p. 11.

32 *Menstrual periods:* American Cancer Society, "Breast Cancer Facts and Figures 2009–2010," p. 12.

33 *Number of births:* Ibid. Rosner B, Colditz GA, Willett WC. "Reproductive risk factors in a prospective study of breast cancer: The Nurses' Health Study." *American Journal of Epidemiology.* 1994;139:819–835.

33 *Birth control pills:* American Cancer Society, "Breast Cancer Facts and Figures 2009–2010," p. 12. Collaborative Group on Hormonal Factors in Breast Cancer. "Breast cancer and hormonal contraceptives: Collaborative reanalysis of individual data on 53,297 women with breast cancer and 100,239 women without breast cancer from 54 epidemiological studies." *Lancet.* 1996;347:1713–1727. Hankinson SE, Colditz GA, Hunter DJ, Spencer TL, Rosner B, Stampfer MJ. "A quantitative assessment of oral contraceptive use and risk of ovarian cancer." *Obstetrics and Gynecology.* 1992;80(4):708–714. Emons G, Fleckenstein G, Hinney B, Huschmand A, Heyl W. "Hormonal interactions in endometrial cancer." *Endocrine-Related Cancer.* 2000;7(4):227–242. National Cancer Institute, "Oral contraceptives and cancer risk: Questions and answers." www.cancer.gov.

33 *Hormone replacement therapy:* Heiss G, Wallace R, Anderson GL, Aragaki A, Beresford SA, Brzyski R, Chlebowski RT, Gass M, LaCroix A, Manson JE, Prentice RL, Rossouw J, Stefanick ML, WHI Investigators. "Health risks and benefits 3 years after stopping randomized treatment with estrogen and progestin." *Journal of the American Medical Association.* 2008 Mar 5;299(9):1036–1045.

34 *Breast-feeding:* American Cancer Society, "Detailed Guide: Breast Cancer: What are the risk factors for breast cancer?" www.cancer.org. Collaborative Group on Hormonal Factors in Breast Cancer. "Breast cancer and breastfeeding: Collaborative reanalysis of individual data from 47 epidemiological studies in 30 countries, including 50,302 women with breast cancer and 96,973 women without the disease." *Lancet.* 2002 Jul 20;360(9328):187–195.

34 *Being Overweight:* Feigelson HS, Jonas CR, Teras LR, Thun MJ, Calle EE. "Weight gain, body mass index, hormone replacement therapy, and post-

menopausal breast cancer in a large prospective study." *Journal of Cancer Epidemiology Biomarkers and Prevention.* 2004 Feb 1;13:220–222.

34 *Physical activity:* McTiernan A, Kooperberg C, White E, Wilcox S, Coates R, Adams-Campbell LL, Woods N, Ockene J. "Recreational physical activity and the risk of breast cancer in postmenopausal women: The Women's Health Initiative cohort study." *Journal of the American Medical Association.* 2003;290:1331–1336.

35 *Alcohol:* Singletary KW, Gapstur SM. "Alcohol and breast cancer: Review of epidemiologic and experimental evidence and potential mechanisms." *Journal of the American Medical Association.* 2001 Nov 7;286(17):2143–2151. Allen NE, Beral V, Casabonne D, Kan SW, Reeves GK, Brown A, Green J, Million Women Study Collaborators. "Moderate alcohol intake and cancer incidence in women." *Journal of the National Cancer Institute.* 2009 Mar 4;101(5):296–305. Pub. online 2009 Feb 24. American Cancer Society, "Detailed Guide: Breast Cancer: What are the risk factors for breast cancer?" www.cancer.org.

CHAPTER FOUR. TO TEST OR NOT TO TEST

45 *increased risk for ovarian cancer . . . a second breast cancer:* Malone KE, Begg CB, Halle RW, Borg A, Concannon P, Tellhed L, Xue S, Teraoka S, Bernstein L, Capanu M, Reiner AS, Riedel ER, Thomas DC, Mellemkjaer L, Lynch CF, Boice JD, Jr., Anton-Culver M, Bernstein JL, "Population-based study of the risk of second primary contralateral breast cancer associated with carrying a mutation in BRCA1 or BRCA2." *Journal of Clinical Oncology.* Pub. online 5 April 2010, ahead of print. Robson M, Svahn T, McCormick B, Borgen P, Hudis CA, Norton L, Offit K. "Appropriateness of breast-conserving treatment of breast carcinoma in women with germline mutations in BRCA1 or BRCA2." *Cancer.* 2005 Jan 1;103(1):44–51.

47 *thousands of possible mutations:* Author interviews with Rebecca Sutphen, M.D., 2009.

47 *which in women indicates up to an 87 percent lifetime chance . . . and up to a 44 percent lifetime chance:* Ford D, Easton DF, Bishop DT, Narod SA, Goldgar DE. "Risks of cancer in BRCA1-mutation carriers. Breast Cancer Linkage Consortium." *Lancet.* 1994 Mar 19;343(8899):692–695.

CHAPTER FIVE. WEIGHING THE OPTIONS: NONSURGICAL

59 *the five-year survival rate for women:* American Cancer Society, "Breast Cancer Facts and Figures 2009–2010," p. 9.

62 *a major national trial found that while digital mammograms have no benefit:* Pisano E, Gatsonis C, Hendrick E, Yaffe M, Baum J, Acharyya S, Conant E, Fajardo L, Bassett L, D'Orsi C, Jong R, Rebner M. "Diagnostic performance of digital

versus film mammography for breast cancer screening—The results of the American College of Radiology Imaging Network (ACRIN) Digital Mammographic Imaging Screening Trial (DMIST)." *New England Journal of Medicine.* Pub. online 15 Sept and in print 27 Oct 2005.

64 *MRI . . . extremely sensitive . . . don't pick up . . . lead to false positives:* Bluemke DA, Gatsonis CA, Chen MH, DeAngelis GA, DeBruhl N, Harms S, Heywang-Kobrunner SH, Hylton N, Kuhl CK, Lehman C, Pisano ED, Causer P, Schnitt SJ, Smazal SF, Stelling CB, Weatherall PT, Schnall MD. "Magnetic resonance imaging of the breast prior to biopsy." *Journal of the American Medical Association.* 2004;292(22):2735–2742.

64 *One study by the American College of Radiology Imaging Network:* Berg W, Blume J, Cormack J, Mendelson E, Lehrer D, Böhm-Vélez M, Pisano E, Jong R, Evans WP, Morton M. "Combined screening with ultrasound and mammography compared to mammography alone: Results of the first-year screen in ACRIN 6666." *Journal of the American Medical Association.* 2008 May;299(18):2151–2163.

65 *Many breast-imaging centers now have computer programs:* Freer TW, Ulissey MJ. "Screening mammography with computer-aided detection: Prospective study of 12,860 patients in a community breast center." *Radiology.* 2001 Sept;220(3):781–786.

65 *others have found that it increases the false-positive rate:* Fenton JJ, Taplin SH, Carney PA, Abraham L, Sickles EA, D'Orsi C, Berns EA, Cutter G, Hendrick RE, Barlow WE, Elmore JG. "Influence of computer-aided detection on performance of screening mammography." *New England Journal of Medicine.* 2007 Apr 5; 356(14):1399–1409. National Cancer Institute, "Computer-aided detection reduces the accuracy of mammograms." www.cancer.gov.

66 *If ovarian cancer is found early and treated:* Ovarian Cancer National Alliance statistics: http://www.ovariancancer.org/about-ovarian-cancer/statistics/.

66 *one woman in seventy-one gets the disease during her lifetime:* Ibid.

68 *when results from a national study showed that women are 49 percent:* Vogel VG, Costantino JP, et. al., for the National Surgical Adjuvant Breast and Bowel Project (NSABP). "Effects of tamoxifen vs raloxifene on the risk of developing invasive breast cancer and other disease outcomes: The NSABP study of tamoxifen and raloxifene (STAR) P-2 Trial." *Journal of the American Medical Association.* 2006;295:2727–2741. Pub. online 5 Jun 2006. Long-term follow-up results of this study were presented at the American Association for Cancer Research (AACR) annual meeting, Washington, D.C., April 17–21, 2010.

68 *Side effects of tamoxifen and raloxifene:* Land SR, Wickerham DL, et.al. "Patient-reported symptoms and quality of life during treatment with tamoxifen or raloxifene for breast cancer prevention: The NSABP study of tamoxifen

and raloxifene (STAR) P-2 Trial." *Journal of the American Medical Association.* 2006;295:2742–2751. Pub. online 5 Jun 2006. Long-term follow-up results of this study were presented at the American Association for Cancer Research (AACR) annual meeting, Washington, D.C., April 17–21, 2010.

70 *Studies have shown that taking birth control pills for five or more years:* Hankinson SE, Colditz GA, Hunter DJ, Spencer TL, Rosner B, Stampfer MJ. "A quantitative assessment of oral contraceptive use and risk of ovarian cancer." *Obstetrics and Gynecology.* 1992;80(4):708–714. Narod SA, Risch H, Moslehi R, Neuhausen S, Moller P, Olsson H, Provencher D, Radice P, Evans G, Bishop S, Brunet JS, Easton D, Hereditary Ovarian Cancer Clinical Study Group. "Oral contraceptive use reduces the risk of hereditary ovarian cancer." *New England Journal of Medicine.* 1998;339:424–428.

70 *other studies conflict over whether or not this benefit applies:* Modan B, Hartge P, Hirsh-Yechezkel G, Chetrit A, Lubin F, Beller U, Ben-Baruch G, Fishman A, Menczer J, Struewing JP, Tucker MA, Wacholder S, National Israel Ovarian Cancer Study Group. "Parity, oral contraceptives, and the risk of ovarian cancer among carriers and noncarriers of a BRCA1 or BRCA2 mutation." *New England Journal of Medicine.* 2001 Jul 26;345(4):235–240. Whittemore AS, Balise RR, Pharoah PD, Dicioccio RA, Oakley-Girvan I, Ramus SJ, Daly M, Usinowicz MB, Garlinghouse-Jones K, Ponder BA, Buys S, Senie R, Andrulis I, John E, Hopper JL, Piver MS. "Oral contraceptive use and ovarian cancer risk among carriers of BRCA1 or BRCA2 mutations." *British Journal of Cancer.* 2004 Nov 29;91(11):1911–1915.

70 *Oral contraceptives may increase the odds:* American Cancer Society, "Breast Cancer Facts and Figures 2009–2010," p. 12. Collaborative Group on Hormonal Factors in Breast Cancer. "Breast cancer and hormonal contraceptives: Collaborative reanalysis of individual data on 53,297 women with breast cancer and 100,239 women without breast cancer from 54 epidemiological studies." *Lancet.* 1996;347:1713–1727.

CHAPTER SIX. WEIGHING THE OPTIONS: SURGICAL

74 *a bilateral prophylactic mastectomy... can reduce a woman's risk:* Hartmann LC, Schaid DJ, Woods JE, Crotty TP, Myers JL, Arnold PG, Petty PM, Sellers TA, Johnson JL, McDonnell SK, Frost MH, Jenkins RB. "Efficacy of bilateral prophylactic mastectomy in women with a family history of breast cancer." *New England Journal of Medicine.* 1999 Jan 14;340(2):77–84. Hartmann LC, Sellers TA, Schaid DJ, Frank TS, Soderberg CL, Sitta DL, Frost MH, Grant CS, Donohue JH, Woods JE, McDonnell SK, Vockley CW, Deffenbaugh A, Couch FJ, Jenkins RB. "Efficacy of bilateral prophylactic mastectomy

in BRCA1 and BRCA2 gene mutation carriers." *Journal of the National Cancer Institute.* 2001 Nov;93(21):1633–1637.

77 *women should at least know that nipple sparing is available:* Rusby JE, Smith BL, Gui GP. "Nipple-sparing mastectomy." *British Journal of Surgery* 2010 Mar;97(3):305–316. Sacchini V, Pinotti JA, Barros AC, Luini A, Pluchinotta A, Pinotti M, Boratto MG, Ricci MD, Ruiz CA, Nisida AC, Veronesi P, Petit J, Arnone P, Bassi F, Disa JJ, Garcia-Etienne CA, Borgen PI. "Nipple-sparing mastectomy for breast cancer and risk reduction: Oncologic or technical problem?" *Journal of the American College of Surgeons* 2006 Nov;203(5):704–714. Pub. online 2006 Sept 11. Gerber B, Krause A, Dieterich M, Kundt G, Reimer T. "The oncological safety of skin sparing mastectomy with conservation of the nipple-areola complex and autologous reconstruction: An extended follow-up study." *Annals of Surgery.* 2009 Mar;249(3):461–468. Voltura AM, Tsangaris TN, Rosson GD, Jacobs LK, Flores JI, Singh NK, Argani P, Balch CM. "Nipple-sparing mastectomy: Critical assessment of 51 procedures and implications for selection criteria." *Annals of Surgical Oncology.* 2008 Dec;15(12):3396–3401. Pub. online 2008 Oct 16.

84 *This operation reduces these women's chances:* Rebbeck TR, Kauff ND, Domchek SM. "Meta-analysis of risk reduction estimates associated with risk-reducing salpingo-oophorectomy in BRCA1 or BRCA2 mutation carriers." *Journal of the National Cancer Institute.* 2009 Jan 21;101(2):80–87. Pub. online 2009 Jan 13.

CHAPTER SEVEN. MONEY MATTERS

94 *Genetic counseling session: About $100–$200:* Author interviews with Angela Trepanier, past president of the National Society of Genetic Counselors, 2009.

94 *The cost of a BRACAnalysis test:* Myriad Genetics, 2009.

94 *Screening mammogram: $80 to $150:* Low end according to the American College of Radiology and the 2008 costs as determined by the Centers for Medicare & Medicaid Services. High end based on costs at medical centers throughout the United States.

94 *Screening digital mammogram: $130 to $250:* Low end according to the American College of Radiology and the 2008 costs as determined by the Centers for Medicare & Medicaid Services. High end based on costs at medical centers throughout the United States.

94 *Breast ultrasound: $80 to $175:* Low end according to the American College of Radiology and the 2008 costs as determined by the Centers for Medicare & Medicaid Services. High end based on costs at medical centers throughout the United States.

94 *Breast MRI: $850 to $2,000:* Low end according to the American College of Radiology and the 2008 costs as determined by the Centers for Medicare & Medicaid Services. High end based on costs at medical centers throughout the United States.

94 *Raloxifene ... about $125:* According to MS&L, public relations firm for Eli Lilly.

94 *Tamoxifen ... about $40:* Based on prices at various pharmacies throughout the United States.

95 *Bilateral prophylactic mastectomy: Around $1,500 to $8,000 or higher:* Low end reflects Medicare costs. High end based on data from various medical centers throughout the United States.

95 *Reconstruction: $2,500 to $25,000 or higher:* Low end reflects Medicare costs. High end based on data from various medical centers throughout the United States.

95 *Nipple reconstruction: Between $1,200 and $6,000:* Low end reflects Medicare costs. High end based on data from various medical centers throughout the United States.

95 *Nipple tattooing: About $1,000 or less:* Low end reflects Medicare costs. High end based on data from various medical centers throughout the United States.

95 *Oophorectomy: $1,000 or higher:* Low end reflects Medicare costs. High end based on data from various medical centers throughout the United States.

95 *Oophorectomy with hysterectomy: $1,500 or higher:* Low end reflects Medicare costs. High end based on data from various medical centers throughout the United States.

CHAPTER EIGHT. A CONTROVERSIAL DECISION

110 *A study in the* Journal of Clinical Oncology *found:* Tuttle TM, Habermann EB, Grund EH, Morris TJ, Virnig BA. "Increasing use of contralateral prophylactic mastectomy for breast cancer patients: A trend toward more aggressive surgical treatment." *Journal of Clinical Oncology.* 2007 Nov 20;25(33):5203–5209. Pub. online 2007 Oct 22.

117 *the surgery lowers the odds ... by almost 50 percent ... by about 80 percent:* Rebbeck TR, Kauff ND, Domchek SM. "Meta-analysis of risk reduction estimates associated with risk-reducing salpingo-oophorectomy in BRCA1 or BRCA2 mutation carriers." *Journal of the National Cancer Institute.* 2009 Jan 21;101(2):80–87. Pub. online 2009 Jan 13.

119 *women who regret having had a prophylactic mastectomy:* Borgen PI, Hill AD, Tran KN, Van Zee KJ, Massie MJ, Payne D, Biggs CG. "Patient regrets after bilateral prophylactic mastectomy." *Annals of Surgical Oncology.* 1998 Oct-Nov;5(7):603–606.

CHAPTER NINE. DEFUSING THE TIME BOMB:
A STEP-BY-STEP GUIDE TO PROPHYLACTIC SURGERY

121 *two-thirds of women who had had a mastectomy wished:* Rolnick SJ, Altschuler A, Nekhlyudov L, Elmore JG, Greene SM, Harris EL, Herrinton LJ, Barton MB, Geiger AM, Fletcher SW. "What women wish they knew before prophylactic mastectomy." *Cancer Nursing.* 2007 Jul-Aug; 30(4); 285–291.

144 *nearly three-quarters of patients who had the procedure were satisfied:* Frost MH, Schaid DJ, Sellers TA, Slezak JM, Arnold PG, Woods JE, Petty PM, Johnson JL, Sitta DL, McDonnell SK, Rummans TA, Jenkins RB, Sloan JA, Hartmann LC. "Long-term satisfaction and psychological and social function following bilateral prophylactic mastectomy." *Journal of the American Medical Association.* 2000;284:319–324.

144 *100 percent of women who had bilateral prophylactic mastectomies were satisfied:* Spear SL, Schwarz KA, Venturi ML, Barbosa T, Al-Attar A. "Prophylactic mastectomy and reconstruction: Clinical outcomes and patient satisfaction." *Plastic and Reconstructive Surgery.* 2008 July;122(1):1–9.

CHAPTER TEN. LOVE, SEX, AND BABIES

156 *women who tested positive for a genetic mutation were considerably more likely:* Wylie JE, Smith KR, Botkin JR. "Effects of spouses on distress experienced by BRCA1 mutation carriers over time." *American Journal of Medical Genetics.* 2003 May 15;119C(1):35–44.

168 *although 68 percent of the respondents have never heard of PGD:* Quinn G, Vadaparampil S, Wilson C, King L, Choi J, Miree C, Friedman S. "Attitudes of high-risk women toward preimplantation genetic diagnosis." *Fertility and Sterility.* 2009 Jun;91(6):2361–2368.

168 *Further research has shown that while some women felt cheated:* Author interviews with Gwendolyn Quinn, Ph.D., 2009.

CHAPTER ELEVEN. BREAST OBSESSION AND BODY IMAGE

171 *type "breast" into Google and you'll get more than 85 million hits:* Google search, March 15, 2010. "Breast" had 86,200,000 hits; "boobs," 39,700,000.

181 *The most common side effects of raloxifene:* Evista website, April 19, 2010. www. evista.com.

183 *when women who had prophylactic mastectomies were surveyed:* Brandberg Y, Sandelin K, Erikson S, Jurell G, Liljegren A, Lindblom A, Lindén A, von Wachenfeldt A, Wickman M, Arver B. "Psychological reactions, quality of life, and body image after bilateral prophylactic mastectomy in women at high risk for breast cancer: A prospective 1-year follow-up study." *Journal of Clinical Oncology.* 2008 Aug 20;26 (24):3943–3949.

183 *Dr. Frost from the Mayo Clinic also found:* Frost MH, Slezak JM, Tran NV, Williams CI, Johnson JL, Woods JE, Petty PM, Donohue JH, Grant CS, Sloan JA, Sellers TA, Hartmann LC. "Satisfaction after contralateral prophylactic mastectomy: The significance of mastectomy type, reconstructive complications, and body appearance." *Journal of Clinical Oncology.* 2005 Nov 1;23(31):7849–7856.

CHAPTER TWELVE. THE HIDDEN KILLER IN MEN

190 *99 percent of people affected are women:* American Cancer Society, "Breast Cancer Facts and Figures 2009–2010," p. 8.

192 *number-one non-skin cancer among men . . . about 192,000 men . . . one-in-six chance:* Prostate Cancer Foundation, 2009. www.prostatecancerfoundation.org

192 *those with a BRCA2 mutation may have:* Ibid. American Cancer Society, "Breast Cancer Genes Can Affect Men, Too." www.cancer.org.

192 *most cases of prostate cancer occur in men older than sixty-five:* Prostate Cancer Foundation, 2009. www.prostatecancerfoundation.org.

192 *But when a man has a BRCA gene mutation:* FORCE, "Other Cancer Risks." www .facingourrisk.org. Liede A, Karlan B, Narod SA. "Cancer risks for male carriers of germline mutations in BRCA1 or BRCA2: A review of the literature." *Journal of Clinical Oncology.* 2004 Feb 15;22(4):735–742.

192 *the chances are 1.2 percent . . . and 6.8 percent:* Chuan Tai Y, Domchek S, Parmigiani G, Chen S. "Breast cancer risk among male BRCA1 and BRCA2 Mutation Carriers." *Journal of the National Cancer Institute.* 2007;99(23):1811–1814.

193 *the majority of men are unaware of their risk:* Daly MB. "The impact of social roles on the experience of men in BRCA1/2 families: Implications for counseling." *Journal of Genetic Counseling.* 2009 Feb 18;(1):42–48. Pub. online 2008 Aug 8.

CHAPTER THIRTEEN. A MOTHER'S LEGACY

199 *half of parents with a BRCA mutation told their minor children:* Bradbury AR, Dignam JJ, Ibe CN, Auh SL, Hlubocky FJ, Cummings SA, White M, Olopade OI, Daugherty CK. "How often do BRCA mutation carriers tell their young children of the family's risk for cancer? A study of parental disclosure of BRCA mutations to minors and young adults." *Journal of Clinical Oncology.* 2007 Aug 20;25(24):3705–3711.

200 *children as young as four getting tested:* "Debate rises over testing children for breast cancer gene." *State Journal Register* (Springfield, IL). Pub. online 27 Oct 2008. www.sj-r.com/features/x1348683501/Debate-rises-over-testing-children-for-breast-cancer-gene. "Breast Cancer Gene Tests for Girls: Too Soon?" ABC

News/Health, June 5, 2008. abcnews.go.com/Health/OnCallPlusBreastCan
cerNews/story?id=5001283&page=1.

CHAPTER FOURTEEN. A PROMISING FUTURE

217 *about 70 percent of breast cancers are influenced by environmental factors:* Lichtenstein
P, Holm NV, Verkasalo PK, Iliadou A, Kaprio J, Koskenvuo M, Pukkala E,
Skytthe A, Hemminki K. "Environmental and heritable factors in the causa-
tion of cancer—Analyses of cohorts of twins from Sweden, Denmark, and
Finland." *New England Journal of Medicine.* 2000 Jul 13;343(2):78–85.

217 *among women with BRCA mutations, eating a diversity:* Ghadirian P, Narod S,
Fafard E, Costa M, Robidoux A, Nkondjock A. "Breast cancer risk in rela-
tion to the joint effect of BRCA mutations and diet diversity." *Breast Cancer
Research and Treatment.* 2009 Sept;117(2):417–422. Pub. online 2009 Jan 23.

217 *research to determine the effects exercise can have:* WISER (Women in Steady Exercise Research) sister program, University of Pennsylvania Center for Clinical
Epidemiology and Biostatistics.

218 *the survival rate is higher than 95 percent:* American Cancer Society, "Breast Cancer Facts and Figures 2009–2010," p. 9.

219 *Some studies have found it highly sensitive:* Brem RF, Floerke AC, Rapelyea JA, Teal
C, Kelly T, Mathur V. "Breast-specific gamma imaging as an adjunct imaging
modality for the diagnosis of breast cancer." *Journal of Academic Radiology.* 2008
Jun;247(3):651–657. Brem RF, Fishman M, Rapelyea JA. "Detection of ductal
carcinoma in situ with mammography, breast specific gamma imaging, and
magnetic resonance imaging: A comparative study." *Academic Radiology.* 2007
Aug;14(8):945–950. Brem RF, Ioffe M, Rapelyea JA, Yost KG, Weigert JM,
Bertrand ML, Stern LH. "Invasive lobular carcinoma: Detection with mammography, sonography, MRI, and breast-specific gamma imaging." *American
Journal of Roentgenology.* 2009 Feb;192(2):379–383.

220 *BSGI also appears to have a greater specificity:* Brem RF, Petrovitch I, Rapelyea JA,
Young H, Teal C, Kelly T. "Breast-specific gamma imaging with 99mTc-Sestamibi
and magnetic resonance imaging in the diagnosis of breast cancer—A comparative study." *Breast Journal.* 2007 Sept-Oct;13(5):465–469.

220 *Positron emission mammography (PEM):* "Effect of breast density, menopausal status, and hormone use in high resolution positron emission mammography."
Study results reported at the 94th Scientific Assembly and Annual Meeting
of the Radiological Society of North America, December 2008.

222 *the drug doesn't appear to lower risk:* Author interviews with Leslie Ford, M.D.
King MC, Wieand S, Hale K, Lee M, Walsh T, Owens K, Tait J, Ford L,
Dunn BK, Costantino J, Wickerham L, Wolmark N, Fisher B, National

Surgical Adjuvant Breast and Bowel Project. "Tamoxifen and breast cancer incidence among women with inherited mutations in BRCA1 and BRCA2: National Surgical Adjuvant Breast and Bowel Project (NSABP-P1) Breast Cancer Prevention Trial." *Journal of the American Medical Association.* 2001 Nov 14;286(18):2251–2256.

223 *Early studies of a class of drugs called Parp inhibitors:* Fong PC, Boss DS, Yap TA, Tutt A, Wu P, Mergui-Roelvink M, Mortimer P, Swaisland H, Lau A, O'Connor MJ, Ashworth A, Carmichael J, Kaye SB, Schellens JH, de Bono JS. "Inhibition of poly(ADP-ribose) polymerase in tumors from BRCA mutation carriers." *New England Journal of Medicine* 2009 Jul 9;361(2):123–134. Pub. online 2009 Jun 24. De Soto JA, Deng CX. "PARP-1 inhibitors: Are they the long-sought genetically specific drugs for BRCA1/2-associated breast cancers?" *International Journal of Medical Sciences* 2006;3:117–123.

226 *under investigation and an option for women:* Clinical trials being conducted by Mentor Corporation, Allergan, and Sientra.

227 *birth control pills are still the most effective medication used to prevent ovarian cancer:* Hankinson SE, Colditz GA, Hunter DJ, Spencer TL, Rosner B, Stampfer MJ. "A quantitative assessment of oral contraceptive use and risk of ovarian cancer." *Obstetrics and Gynecology* 1992;80(4):708–714. Narod SA, Risch H, Moslehi R, Neuhausen S, Moller P, Olsson H, Provencher D, Radice P, Evans G, Bishop S, Brunet JS, Easton D, Hereditary Ovarian Cancer Clinical Study Group (1998). "Oral contraceptive use reduces the risk of hereditary ovarian cancer." *New England Journal of Medicine,* 339:424–428.

227 *not yet entirely clear whether or not those statistics apply:* Modan B, Hartge P, Hirsh-Yechezkel G, Chetrit A, Lubin F, Beller U, Ben-Baruch G, Fishman A, Menczer J, Struewing JP, Tucker MA, Wacholder S, National Israel Ovarian Cancer Study Group. "Parity, oral contraceptives, and the risk of ovarian cancer among carriers and noncarriers of a BRCA1 or BRCA2 mutation." *New England Journal of Medicine.* 2001 Jul 26;345(4):235–240. Whittemore AS, Balise RR, Pharoah PD, Dicioccio RA, Oakley-Girvan I, Ramus SJ, Daly M, Usinowicz MB, Garlinghouse-Jones K, Ponder BA, Buys S, Senie R, Andrulis I, John E, Hopper JL, Piver MS. "Oral contraceptive use and ovarian cancer risk among carriers of BRCA1 or BRCA2 mutations." *British Journal of Cancer.* 2004 Nov 29;91(11):1911–1915.

228 *Preliminary results show promise:* Author interview with David Fishman, M.D., 2009.

resources

- FORCE (www.facingourrisk.org)
- Bright Pink (www.bebrightpink.org)
- Sharsheret (www.sharsheret.org)
- Jacob International (www.jacobintl.org)
- Power of Pink (www.thepowerofpinkfl.com)
- Think Pink Rocks (www.thinkpinkrocks.org)

GENERAL INFORMATION ABOUT CANCER
- American Cancer Society (www.cancer.org)
- Susan G. Komen for the Cure (ww5.komen.org)
- National Cancer Institute (www.cancer.gov)
- Breast Cancer Research Foundation (www.bcrfcure.org)
- Young Survival Coalition (www.youngsurvival.org)
- Stand Up To Cancer (www.standup2cancer.org)
- Breast Cancer Network of Strength (www.networkofstrength.org)
- Breastcancer.org: A comprehensive resource that provides information about the disease (www.breastcancer.org).

RISK ASSESSMENT AND GENETICS
- National Society of Genetic Counselors (www.nsgc.org)
- Myriad Genetic Laboratories (www.myriad.com)
- National Cancer Institute (www.cancer.gov/search/geneticsservices)
- Informed Medical Decisions (www.informeddna.com)
- Gail Model (www.cancer.gov/bcrisktool)

- Genetic Alliance (www.geneticalliance.org)
- National Human Genome Research Institute (www.genome.gov)
- American Society of Human Genetics (www.ashg.org)

INSURANCE AND FINANCIAL ASSISTANCE

- Patient Advocate Foundation (www.patientadvocate.org)
- National Breast and Cervical Cancer Early Detection Program (www.cdc.gov/cancer/NBCCEDP)
- Myriad (www.myriadtests.com)
- Partnership for Prescription Assistance (www.pparx.org)
- Right Action for Women (www.rightactionforwomen.org)

FINDING MULTIDISCIPLINARY CENTERS

- National Cancer Institute (www.cancer.gov)
- FORCE (www.facingourrisk.org)
- Association of Community Cancer Centers (www.accc-cancer.org)
- National Consortium of Breast Centers (www.breastcare.org)
- National Comprehensive Cancer Network (www.nccn.org/members/network.asp)

FINDING DOCTORS

- American Society of Breast Surgeons (www.breastsurgeons.org)
- Society of Surgical Oncology (www.surgonc.org)
- American Society of Plastic Surgeons (www.plasticsurgery.org)
- American Congress (College) of Obstetricians and Gynecologists (www.acog.org)
- Society of Gynecologic Oncologists (www.sgo.org)

INFORMATION ABOUT OVARIAN CANCER AND SURGICAL SUPPORT

- Ovarian Cancer National Alliance (www.ovariancancer.org)
- Ovarian Cancer Institute (www.ovariancancerinstitute.org)
- HysterSisters (www.hystersisters.com)

CLINICAL TRIALS AND RESEARCH

- National Cancer Institute (www.cancer.gov/clinicaltrials/search)
- National Institutes of Health (clinicaltrials.gov)
- American College of Radiology Imaging Network (www.acrin.org)
- Army of Women (www.armyofwomen.org)

MENTAL HEALTH SUPPORT
- American Psychological Association (www.apa.org)
- American Association of Sexuality Educators, Counselors and Therapists (www.aasect.org)

BREAST RECONSTRUCTION PHOTOS AND INFORMATION
- My Breast Reconstruction (www.mybreastreconstruction.com)
- Center for Restorative Breast Surgery (www.breastcenter.com)
- The Center for Microsurgical Breast Reconstruction (www.diepflap.com)
- *The Breast Reconstruction Guidebook* by Kathy Steligo (www.breastrecon.com)
- FORCE (www.facingourrisk.org)

OTHER RESOURCES
- *Previvors* official book website (www.previvors.com)
- *Previvors* official author website (www.dinarothport.com)
- *Pretty Is What Changes* by Jessica Queller (www.jessicaqueller.com)
- *In the Family* documentary (inthefamily.kartemquin.com)
- Breast Self-Exam Tool (ww5.komen.org/BreastCancer/InteractiveTools .html)

index